SIRTFOOD DIET

And

MEDITERRANEAN DIET COOKBOOK FOR BEGINNERS

2 in 1 Bundle

G.S. Van Lee

Disclaimer

The information contained in " SIRTFOOD DIET AndMEDITERRANEAN DIET COOKBOOK FOR BEGINNERS2 in 1 Bundleis meant to serve as a comprehensive collection of strategies that the author of this eBook has done research about. Summaries, strategies, tips and tricks are only recommendation by the author, and reading this eBook will not guarantee that one's results will exactly mirror the author's results. The author of the eBook has made all reasonable effort to provide current and accurate information for the readers of the eBook. The author and it's associates will not be held liable for any unintentional error or omissions that may be found. The material in the eBook may include information by third parties. Third party materials comprise of opinions expressed by their owners. As such, the author of the eBook does not assume responsibility or liability for any third party material or opinions. Whether because of the progression of the internet, or the unforeseen changes in company policy and editorial submission guidelines, what is stated as fact at the time of this writing may become autdated or inapplicable later.

The eBook is copyright © 2020 with all rights reserved. It is illegal to redistribute , copy, or create derivative work from this eBook whole or in part. No parts of this report may be reproduced or retransmitted in any reproduced or retransmitted in any forms whatsoever without the writing expressed and signed permission from the author.

Sommario

Introduction 18

What Is Sirtfood? 19

How the Sirrfood Diet Works 21

The first stage of the diet 22

The second stage of the diet 22

After the diet, ... 23

Is It Effective? 23

How to Follow the Sirtfood Diet 26

Sirtfood Meal Plan and 3 Weeks Plan 28

Meal Planning 33

THE SIRRFOOD DIET RECIPES   36

1. RABBIT WITH APPLES 36
2. HUNGARIAN APPLE PIE 37
3. SIMILY SISTERS APPLE PIE 39
4. WULFS APPLE PIE 40
5. ALSATIAN APPLE PIE 41
6. SEMOLINA APPLE PIE 44
7. PROVENCAL APPLE PIE WITH WALNUTS 45
8. WARSAW APPLE PIE 46

9.	SIMPLE APPLE PIE	48
10.	Sand Cheese And Apple Pie	50
11.	DORADO WITH CITRUS PESTO SAUCE	51
12.	CITRUS JAM	53
13.	CITRUS CURD CASSEROLE	53
14.	BLUEBERRY CITRUS SMOOTHIE	54
15.	COCKTAIL OF THREE TYPES OF CITRUS WITH MAPLE SYRUP	55
16.	QUINOA, SHRIMP AND CITRUS SALAD	56
17.	CITRUS MIX PUDDING	57
18.	CARROT SALAD WITH CITRUS MARINADE WITH CHANAH CHEESE	60
19.	ORANGE CITRUS AND PERSIMMON SALAD	61
20.	MANNIK COTTAGE CHEESE "STRAWBERRIES WITH CREAM"	63
21.	PUMPKIN CITRUS DESSERT	64
22.	"LEMONADE" FROM…. CUCUMBERS	65
23.	PINEAPPLE - CITRUS SORBET WITH LIQUOR	66
24.	MULLED WINE	67
25.	CHRISTMAS MULLED WINE	68
26.	NON-ALCOHOLIC MULLED WINE	70
27.	MULLED WINE WITH COFFEE AND COGNAC	70
28.	FRUIT MULLED WINE	71
29.	CHRISTMAS MULLED WINE WITH WHITE WINE AND ORANGES	72

30.	WINTER MULLED WINE	73
31.	BUCKWHEAT MEATBALLS WITH MUSHROOMS	74
32.	BUCKWHEAT CHICKEN CUTLETS	77
33.	BUCKWHEAT DIET CUTLETS	78
34.	BUCKWHEAT CUTLETS	79
35.	BUCKWHEAT AND COTTAGE CHEESE CUTLETS	81
36.	MEATBALLS WITH BUCKWHEAT IN A SLOW COOKER	82
37.	BUCKWHEAT CUTLETS (LEAN)	84
38.	MEATBALLS WITH BUCKWHEAT AND MINCED MEAT	85
39.	BUCKWHEAT AND MINCED MEATBALLS	86
40.	VEGETARIAN CUTLETS WITH BUCKWHEAT AND POTATOES	89
41.	EGGPLANT WITH WALNUT AND GARLIC	90
42.	RED BEAN LOBIO	91
43.	GEORGIAN EGGPLANT WITH NUTS	92
44.	COOKIES "CIGARETTES" WITH NUTS	95
45.	LUXURIOUS COOKIES	96
46.	COOKIES "MAZURKA" WITH WALNUTS AND RAISINS	97
47.	ABKHAZIAN EGGPLANT	99

48.nPUFF PASTRY ROLL WITH APPLES 101

49. STRING BEAN SALAD WITH WALNUTS 103

50. BANANA CRUMBLE 106

51. BROWNIES WITH MILK AND DARK CHOCOLATE 107

52. BROWNIE WITH BANANA AND DARK CHOCOLATE........................108

53. VANILLA BROWNIE WITH WALNUTS AND DARK CHOCOLATE 109

54. BROWNIES WITH WALNUTS AND DARK CHOCOLATE 110

55. HOT CHOCOLATE WITH VANILLA AND DARK CHOCOLATE.................113

56. DARK CHOCOLATE CURD CAKE...114

57. DARK CHOCOLATE BROWNIE IN A PAN 115

58. SEMOLINA PORRIDGE WITH WHITE AND DARK CHOCOLATE AND DRIED CHERRY..116

59. STRAWBERRY IN DARK CHOCOLATE WITH WHITE PATTERNS 117

60. CLASSIC BROWNIE WITH DARK CHOCOLATE AND NUTS.........................118

61. LAZY PARSLEY AND PARMESAN SALAD 120

62. UNSWEETENED PIE WITH TOMATOES AND PARSLEY 121

63. VEGETABLE PIE WITH PARSLEY PESTO......................................122

64. CABBAGE SOUP WITH CHICKEN 125

65. BLACK COD CONFIT WITH PARSLEY SALAD.................................126

66. SLOW COOKED FISH SOUP WITH PARSLEY, POTATOES AND CORN 127

67. CARROT SALAD WITH NUTS AND PARSLEY..................................129

68. CHEESE AND PARSLEY PIE 130

69. PARSLEY WITH GARLIC 132

70. YOUNG POTATOES WITH GARLIC AND PARSLEY 133

71. SALSA VERDE WITH PARSLEY AND MINT 135

72. TOMATOES STUFFED WITH SALMON AND CAPERS 135

73. SALAD WITH TUNA AND CAPERS 137

74. SALMON TARTARE WITH CAPERS 137

75. FLOUNDER WITH CAPER AND LEMON OIL 138

76. PASTA WITH TUNA AND CAPERS 140

78. TOMATO SALAD WITH CAPERS 141

79. NICOISE SALAD WITH FRESH TUNA, CAPERS AND ANCHOVIES 142

80. SALMON CARPACCIO WITH CAPERS 144

81. PEPPERS STUFFED WITH TUNA AND CAPERS 145

82. VINAIGRETTE WITH CAPERS AND BAKED BEETS 145

83. SALMON AND CAPER TARTARE 147

84. SPAGHETTI WITH ANCHOVIES, PARSLEY, OLIVES AND CAPERS 148

85. BLUEBERRY PIE 149

86. COTTAGE CHEESE CASSEROLE WITH BLUEBERRIES 151

87. BLUEBERRY MUFFINS 151

88. BLUEBERRY YOGURT BANANA SMOOTHIE 153

89. BLUEBERRY AND CINNAMON MUFFINS 153

90. BLUEBERRY DUMPLINGS 155

91. OATMEAL WITH BANANA AND BLUEBERRIES 157

92. BLUEBERRIES WITH COTTAGE CHEESE AND HONEY 158

93. CHOCOLATE CAKE WITH BLUEBERRIES AND CHERRIES 158

94. BLUEBERRY AND BANANA SMOOTHIE 160

95. TURMERIC LENTIL SOUP 162

96. TURMERIC AND BASIL CARROT PUREE 164

97. STRAWBERRY MOUSSE CURD CAKE 165

98. JELLY CANDIES 167

99. PIE "STRAWBERRY DELIGHT" 170

100. STRAWBERRY CAKE "CLOUD" 171

101. Strawberry Curd Cupcakes 173

102. Strawberry Sponge Cake 175

103. SALAD WITH STRAWBERRIES, MOZZARELLA AND ARUGULA 177

104. STRAWBERRY JAM TART 178

105. STRAWBERRY BANANA SMOOTHIE 180

106. Creamy Strawberry cup 181

107. Apple Green Ceviche 183

108. Soup 'green 185

109. Stuffed Zucchini 187

110. Pumpkins with Quinoa 190

111. Pea salad, gourmet peas, grapefruit 192

112. Indian pea dip 194

113. Millet veggie kale Paupiettes, apple pear chutney 196

114.	Broad beans, peas, gourmet peas and mint	198
115.	Broccoli, Zucchini & Onions Soup: Super Healthy Recipe	200
116.	Irish coffee	202
117.	Caramel coffee	204
118.	Latte macchiato	205
119.	Latte Macchiato Caramel	206
120.	Coffee Cream With Caramel Milk Foam	209
121.	Hot And Cold Vanilla Espresso With Caramel Foam And Cookies	212
122.	Espresso With Cottage Cheese, Lime And Brazil Nuts	215
123.	Coffee with Malice	217
124.	Viennese coffee	218
125.	Coffee mousse	219
126.	Detoxifying milkshake	221
127.	Green pineapple smoothie	222
128.	Chile Campana Smoothie	224
129.	Pumpkin Smoothie in a Glass	226
130.	Berry and Beet Smoothie	228
131.	Pumpkin Spread Cream	230
132.	Chilling raspberry	232
133.	Popeye's Powerful Smoothie	234
134.	Smoothie ananas plant infusion	236

135.	Lemon cream	239
136.	Grouper in green sauce	239
137.	Pumpkin and apple soup	241
138.	Double melon mojito	244
139.	Basil and blackberry mojito	246
140.	Tart apple and carrots soup	248
141.	Black bean and avocado soup	248
142.	Cream of pear and arugula	250
143.	Soup 'green	253
144.	Greek chicken stew with slow cooker	256
145.	Southwestern Chicken Chili Cooked In Slow Cooker	258

SIRTFOOD SNACKS   260

146.	Sand Cheese And Apple Pie	260
147.	COTTAGE CHEESE "STRAWBERRIES WITH CREAM"	262
148.	WINTER MULLED WINE	263
149.	BANANA CRUMBLE	265
150.	STRAWBERRY CAKE "CLOUD"	266

Are Sirtfoods The New Superfoods? 269

Is It Healthy and Sustainable 269

Safety and Side Effects 270

Conclusion 272

INTRODUCTION   275

CHAPTER ONE   278

Understanding the Mediterranean diet 278

What is the Mediterranean diet 279

History of the Mediterranean diet 281

The Science behind the Mediterranean Diet 285

How does the Mediterranean diet work? 286

CHAPTER TWO   288

Living longer with a Mediterranean diet 288

Health Benefits of the Mediterranean Diet 290
   1. Lower risk of heart disease 290
   2. Lower risk of having diabetes 291
   3. Prevents hypertension 291
   4. Prevents fatty liver disease 292
   5. A potentially longer lifespan 292
   6. Improvement of cognitive function 293
   7. Lower risk of cancer 293
   8. Reduction of preservatives and chemicals 294
   9. Increased consumption of antioxidants 294
   10. Less likely to suffer from Parkinson's disease 295

Losing Weight with the Mediterranean Diet 295

CHAPTER THREE   297

Starting the Mediterranean Diet 297

CHAPTER FOUR   300

Eat Well and Stay Healthy the Mediterranean Way 300

Adopting a Mediterranean Style Diet 301

CHAPTER FIVE 311

Mediterranean Diet Food Pyramid Vs Traditional Food Pyramid 311

How to Implement the Mediterranean Diet into Your Lifestyle 314

CHAPTER SIX 317

Reasons Why a Mediterranean Diet in the 21st Century Is A Healthy Choice. 317

A weekly menu based on the Mediterranean diet 320

CHAPTER SEVEN 324

Mediterranean breakfast recipes 324
- Scrambled eggs with truffles 324
- Spaghettiomelett 324
- Croque Monsieur 325
- Crab choux 326
- Greek yogurt with honeycomb 327
- Tramezzini with egg and anchovies 328
- Herb omelet 329
- Caprese Toast 330
- Italian rolls ("pane arabo") 331
- Eggs alla Saltimbocca 332
- Oatmeal Seasoned with Vegetables 333
- Millo and flaxseed pancakes 334
- Millet and buckwheat muffins with black currants 335

Apple and pumpkin pie 337
- Pumpkin and oatmeal bars 338
- Blackberry and lemon muffins for tea 339
- Cocoa, banana, and whole-grain spelled flour muffins 340

Oatmeal and Apple Muffins 341

- Pear and hazelnut crostini 343
- Feta and olive pancakes with bird salad 343

Bruschetta with mozzarella 345

- Greek omelet 346
- Masabacha green lentil curry 347
- Mushroom olive frittata 349
- Broccoli-cheddar quiche with a sweet potato crust 350
- Zucchini and oatmeal muffins 352

CHAPTER EIGHT   355

Mediterranean lunch recipes **355**

- Garden fresh omelets 355
- Mediterranean chicken panini 356

Spinach Stuffed Mushrooms 358
Crispy Cauliflower Chips 360
Baked potatoes without oil 361

- Red cranberry and kale pilaf 361
- Sweet potato tropical casserole 363
- Traditional stuffing 363
- Quinoa Pilaf Stuffing 364
- Mashed sweet potato with cauliflower 365
- Brussels sprouts caramelized with blueberries. 366

Mediterranean chicken with 4 kinds of cheese 367
Mediterranean beef casserole 368
Mediterranean rolls 370
Mediterranean fish fillet 371
Baked fish Mediterranean style 372
Beef Meatballs in Vegetable Bath 373

- Burritos of Cabbage 375
- Black Bean and Quinoa Burgers 377

Roasted Cauliflower with Turmeric 378

- Creamy mushroom lasagna, gluten-free 379

Traditional Greek salad 381
Tomato and feta salad 382
Colorful layered salad 383

- Nopal Soup 384
- Matzo Ball Soup 386

13

CHAPTER NINE   389

Mediterranean dinner recipes 389
- Mediterranean Baked Cod Recipe with Lemon and Garlic 389
- Chicken Shawarma 390
- Moroccan vegetable tagine recipe 392
- Green salad with Chicken Rey and egg 394
- Panera Bread Green Goddess Cobb Salad 395
- Caprese tomato, mozzarella, basil and avocado salad recipe 397
- Creamy Potato Salad 398
- Wedge Salad with Creamy Dressing 399
- Tomatoes stuffed with tuna 400

Seafood paella recipe 402
- Spaghetti and Meatballs 404

Oatmeal Seasoned with Vegetables 406
Rice with Smoked Sausages and Beer 407

CHAPTER TEN   409

Mediterranean dessert recipes 409
- Italian apple and olive oil cake 409

Chocolate Panna Cotta 411
Drunk chocolate cake with mousse and strawberries 412
- crunchy quinoa bars 414
- Apple and pumpkin pie 415
- Blueberry muffins 416
- Brownie Fat Bombs 417
- chocolate Custard 418
- Chocolate Cake Espresso 419
- Chocolate Orange Cupcake 421
- Coconut Ice Cream with Berries 422
- Cranberry Low Carb Cookies 423
- Cherry and poppy seed muffins 424
- Homemade granola 426
- Tofu cashew cheesecake dessert 426
- Christmas nut cake with ginger 428

CHAPTER ELEVEN — 431

Mediterranean snacks recipes 431
- Grilled scallop top in cherry salmorejo 431

Coconut snacks 432

Cucumber and kale open sandwich 433
- Baked zucchini in cheese breading with aioli sauce 435
- Stuffed Eggs with Cheese and Olives 436

Apple "Halloween" lamps 437
- Mediterranean recipe of toasted chickpeas 438
- Bean salad 439
- Spicy red lentil dip. 441
- Coconut Bars with Nuts 441
- Spinach Cheese Bread 442
- Roasted Chickpeas 443
- Almond butter toast with sweet potatoes and blueberries 444

CONCLUSION — 445

SIRTFOOD DIET

The Ultimate Guide For Rapid Weight loss and a Healthy Life. Discovering the incredible benefits of sirtfood that allows you to burn fat like never before.

G.S. Van Leeuwen

Disclaimer

The information contained in " SIRTFOOD DIET is meant to serve as a comprehensive collection of strategies that the author of this eBook has done research about. Summaries, strategies, tips and tricks are only recommendation by the author, and reading this eBook will not guarantee that one's results will exactly mirror the author's results. The author of the eBook has made all reasonable effort to provide current and accurate information for the readers of the eBook. The author and it's associates will not be held liable for any unintentional error or omissions that may be found. The material in the eBook may include information by third parties. Third party materials comprise of opinions expressed by their owners. As such, the author of the eBook does not assume responsibility or liability for any third party material or opinions. Whether because of the progression of the internet, or the unforeseen changes in company policy and editorial submission guidelines, what is stated as fact at the time of this writing may become autdated or inapplicable later.

The eBook is copyright © 2020 with all rights reserved. It is illegal to redistribute , copy, or create derivative work from this eBook whole or in part. No parts of this report may be reproduced or retransmitted in any reproduced or retransmitted in any forms whatsoever without the writing expressed and signed permission from the author.

Introduction

Let's start at the beginning. The Sirtfood diet came to the fore through Instagram - of course. It promises to lose up to 3 kilos a week without eliminating some things that it costs to strike down, chocolate or red wine.

After these first promises, it was also leaked that it is an exclusive diet that was designed for a group of celebrities in one of the most TOP gyms in London that some like Madonna or Daniel Craig go to. Their creators? Renowned Aidan Goggins and Glen Matten, both nutritionists.

What Is Sirtfood?

The Sirtfood diet was developed by two renowned nutritionists working in a private gym in the UK. They advertise the diet as a revolutionary plan for losing weight and improving health, which can trigger changes in the body at the cellular level.

In general, the diet is based on studies of sirtuins, a group of seven proteins found in the body. They regulate various functions, including metabolism, inflammation, and longevity. Some natural plant compounds are able to increase the level of these proteins in the body. And the products containing them received the name "sirfoods" from the authors of the diet.

List of "20 best food" for the Sirtfood diet includes:
- Kale cabbage
- Red wine
- Strawberry
- Bow
- Soybean
- Parsley
- Olive oil
- Dark chocolate (minimum 85% cocoa)
- Japanese matcha green tea
- Buckwheat

- Turmeric
- Walnuts
- Arugula
- Pepper Flame
- Lovage
- Dates Salad chicory
- Blueberries Capers
- Coffee

The diet combines these so-called sweet foods and calorie restriction. Both one and the other, supposedly, can increase the level of sirtuins in the body. The creators of the diet claim that thanks to this, the Sirtfood diet will lead to rapid weight reduction while maintaining muscle mass and protecting against chronic diseases.

How the Sirrfood Diet Works

Sirtfood diet consists of two phases, which last a total of three weeks. After that, you can partially continue the diet by including as many sirfoods as possible in regular dishes. Specific recipes for these two phases are contained in The Sirtfood Diet, written by the creators of the diet. To follow a diet, you have to buy it. However, there are already alternative recipe books and even recipes in the public domain. The bad news is that almost all of them are in various languages. If you do not know the language, you will have to ask someone to translate them.

There may also be a problem with finding all the ingredients necessary for a diet. Matcha and lovage Japanese powdered green tea are not the most popular and affordable products. The most important part of the diet is the juice, which will need to be made one to three times a day. To get this, you need a juicer and a kitchen scale, since the ingredients are measured strictly by weight.

Sirtfood Juice Recipe

- 75 g kale
- 30 grams of arugula
- 5 g parsley
- two sticks of celery
- 1 cm ginger
- Half green apple

- Half a lemon
- Half a teaspoon of matcha green tea powder

All ingredients except green tea and lemon are passed through a juicer and poured into a glass. Lemon juice is squeezed by hand. Then green tea powder is added, and everything is mixed.

The first stage of the diet

The first stage lasts seven days and includes calorie restriction and a lot of juice. At this stage, weight loss starts - in a week, you should lose 3.2 kg. During the first three days of the first phase, calorie intake is limited to 1000 calories per day. You drink three glasses of juice a day, plus one meal. The recipe is selected only from the list allowed for the diet. For example, it can be scrambled eggs or shrimp with buckwheat noodles.

On days 4 through 7, calorie intake rises to 1,500. Now you need to drink two glasses of juice a day and eat two main dishes from the list.

The second stage of the diet

The second stage lasts two weeks, in which you must continue to lose weight. There is no particular calorie limit for this phase. Instead, you eat three main meals a day and drink one glass of juice. Again, dishes are selected from recipes presented in the book or on special sites.

After the diet,

The two phases of the diet can be repeated as often as required for further weight loss. In addition, it is recommended that you continue to add sirfood dishes to your diet even after returning to your normal diet. It is also advised that you continue to drink Sirtfood juice every day. Thus, the Sirtfood diet is more like a lifestyle change than a short-term diet.

Is It Effective?

The authors of the diet make the most daring statements about this. The problem is that there is not enough evidence to support their words. There is no convincing evidence that the Sirtfood diet helps you lose weight more effectively than any other calorie-restricted diet.

Although many of the recommended foods are undoubtedly useful, there have not been any long-term studies in humans that can confirm that overall, such a diet provides tangible health benefits. The original Sirtfood Diet book presents the results of a pilot study conducted by the authors themselves, in which 39 volunteers from the fitness center participated. During the week, participants followed a diet and trained daily. Towards its end, they lost an average of 3.2 kg and retained or even gained muscle mass. But these results are unlikely to surprise anyone. Limiting food intake to 1000 calories a day while doing sports always leads to weight loss. The fact is that when the body is deprived of energy, it uses its reserves, in particular glycogen, in addition to burning fat and muscles. Each glycogen molecule binds 3-4 water molecules in the body. When the body uses glycogen, it also disposes of this water. As a result, we quickly lose weight, but not at the expense of fat. It has been proven that in the first week of extreme calorie restriction, only about one-third of weight loss occurs in fat, while the other two-thirds are water, muscle, and glycogen.

As for calorie intake increases, the body replenishes glycogen stores, and the weight returns. Unfortunately, this kind of calorie restriction can also lead to the fact that the body will reduce the metabolic rate, which will not contribute to further weight loss. That is, probably, the Sirtfood diet can really help to lose a few pounds right at the start, but they will return as soon as the diet is over.

As for the disease prevention promised by the authors, then three weeks is clearly not enough time to seriously affect health. On the other hand, adding sugar foods to your regular diet, in the long run, may well be a good idea. True, in this case, the diet itself can be skipped.

How to Follow the Sirtfood Diet

This nutrition program can be divided into two phases: the so-called march throw (during which you lose excess weight) and fastening. The "march throw" is designed for a week, during which you lose about 3 - 3.5 kg. Having fixed the result, the "march-throw" is repeated - once a month, until the necessary results are obtained. After you gain the weight of your dreams, it is recommended to repeat the "march throw" once every three months.

Get ready to drink plenty of green juice. It is prepared as follows:

2 handfuls of curly cabbage mixed in a blender with a handful of arugula and a handful of parsley, grind into gruel. Add 150 g of celery, including leaves, half a green apple, half lemon juice and a teaspoon of matcha tea powder. Dilute the mixture with still water for a more comfortable drink. Drink this juice should be 1 to 2 hours before meals.

Sirt Food Diet: The First Three Days

The throw march begins. The first three days you need to drink 3 servings of green juice per day and eat one full meal of the recommended (see above) foods. Snacks are also acceptable, but your "limit" of calories is limited to 1000 calories per day.

Sirtfood diet: the next four days

We continue to drink green juice (two servings a day) and allow ourselves two full meals with snacks. Calorie Limit: 1500.

Weight loss at this stage will be 3 - 3.5 kg. If you feel that you can last longer than four days, feel free to continue this diet for another week. The plumb in this case will be even greater.

Sirtfood Diet: Securing Results

For the period of consolidation is not provided for any strict rules. "Just try to include as many "syrfoods "in your diet as possible in order to feel healthier, more energetic and improve the condition of your skin, as well as becoming even slimmer," says Aidan Goggins.

Keep drinking green juice (one serving a day). General recommendations: dinner should be no later than seven o'clock in the evening, exclude processed foods from the diet, reduce the amount of red meat to 500 g per week. Red wine is allowed and even encouraged, but you can drink it no more than 3 times a week.

This phase can last as long as you need. Many who have appreciated the benefits of sirtfood in their experience prefer to build their entire diet on the basis of sirtfoods.

Sirtfood Meal Plan and 3 Weeks Plan

Losing Weight Like Adele: The Sense And Nonsense Of The Sirt Food Diet

Since singer Adele lost tens of kilos with it, the sirt food diet has been in the spotlight. What exactly is sirt food and what are the effects of this diet regime?

Question 1: What is the sirt food diet?

Sirt stands for sirtuin. Foods that contain that substance would stimulate fat burning, improve muscle growth and be good for your health. Examples of sirt foods are cocoa, green tea, walnuts, coffee, turmeric and red onions. British creators Aidan Goggins and Glen Matten, both nutritionists, call the diet "the revolutionary health and weight loss plan." It takes place in two stages. The first week should be the strictest: then you limit yourself to a maximum of two low-calorie meals a day and you mainly drink juices from sirt foods.

This is followed by the maintenance phase: three healthy meals a day for two weeks, one green juice and a maximum of one sirt food snack. You don't eat anything after seven in the evening. After those three weeks, according to the authors, your body gets a fat-burning boost and you lose more than 3 kilos. After this you only have to add a lot of sirtfoods to your diet and possibly repeat the first stages.

Question 2: What do sirtuins do?

"Sirtuins are body's own enzymes, proteins", says Ingeborg Brouwer, professor of nutrition for healthy living at VU University Amsterdam. "The letters 'sir' stands for silent information regulators.

These substances have an important function in our body. They play a role in the regulation of our dna and rna, the genetic material in our cells. They are important in the prevention of cell aging. When you fast, your body produces more sirtuins. This also happens with exercise. The theory is that eating sirt foods has the same effect as fasting and exercising. Among other things, it would increase your metabolism and stimulate fat burning. "

These proteins are indeed in the mentioned foods. But proteins from food are broken down when they are absorbed. They are unlikely to do the same in the body as our body's own enzymes. Whether they cause you to lose weight, I doubt. The sirttfood diet allows you to consume up to 1000 calories in the first three days. Then you lose weight anyway. "

Question 3: Is following this diet heavy?

According to the proponents, it is a piece of cake. The group of foods also has an effect on your brain. The substances are said to regulate hunger via the taste center in your brain. Therefore, you would not feel hungry even in the strictest phase. Since you mimic the effect of exercise with the diet, you don't need to lose yourself in the gym. "The recommended foods fit in well with a healthy diet. You also don't eat too much of it quickly, " says professor Brouwer. Still, there are things to keep in mind. For example, the benefit of chocolate only applies to 85 percent dark chocolate. "Anyone who has ever eaten that knows that the taste is very bitter. The temptation to eat too much is small. "

The weight of the diet also depends on whether it suits you, says Brouwer, who conducts research on diet and depression, among other things. "Not eating after seven in the evening can be a good idea for many people because they consume less, but it has to fit into your life."

Question 4: Are the effects scientifically proven?

Although the diet is 'clinically proven' according to the authors, no large-scale research has been done, Brouwer knows. "Studies with fruit flies and mice have shown that the substances mentioned have beneficial effects, but more research is needed to substantiate the authors' claims."

According to Brouwer, the choice of raw food and fresh products is consistent with the Mediterranean diet, which consists of many fresh vegetables and olive oil. "It has been proven that it contributes to a longer life expectancy and a better quality of life."

Brouwer suspects that the promised weight loss is mainly related to the limited calorie intake. "It's about healthy eating with few calories. In that respect, the diet is not revolutionary. "

Question 5: What if you don't have to lose weight?

Not only superstars swear by the diet plan. Athletes also follow it, because of the beneficial health effects. According to creators Goggins and Matten, a lack of sirtuins in the body plays a role in many diseases, such as diabetes and Alzheimer's disease. Due to its positive effects on muscle building, it would also be good for the heart.

Brouwer: I don't see any major disadvantages. You eat healthy, unprocessed foods and because there are no restrictions on other foods, you do not run out of shortages quickly. Make sure that you do not lose weight with too little or one-sided food. Simply varied, not eating too much and healthy food works best."

Examples of sirtfoods - Dark chocolate (85% cocoa) - Kale - Red onion - Blueberries - Turmeric - Strawberries - Soy - Matcha green tea - Olive oil - Capers - Parsley - Citrus Fruit - Apples - Red praise - Rocket - Walnuts - Buckwheat - Red Wine - Coffee (in moderation)

Meal Planning

This nutrition program can be divided into two phases: the so-called march throw (during which you lose excess weight) and fastening. The "march throw" is designed for a week, during which you lose about 3 - 3.5 kg. Having fixed the result, the "march-throw" is repeated - once a month, until the necessary results are obtained. After you gain the weight of your dreams, it is recommended to repeat the "march throw" once every three months.

Get ready to drink plenty of green juice. It is prepared as follows:

2 handfuls of curly cabbage mixed in a blender with a handful of arugula and a handful of parsley, grind into gruel. Add 150 g of celery, including leaves, half a green apple, half lemon juice and a teaspoon of matcha tea powder. Dilute the mixture with still water for a more comfortable drink. Drink this juice should be 1 to 2 hours before meals.

Sirt Food Diet: The First Three Days

The throw march begins. The first three days you need to drink 3 servings of green juice per day and eat one full meal of the recommended (see above) foods. Snacks are also acceptable, but your "limit" of calories is limited to 1000 calories per day.

Sirtfood diet: the next four days

We continue to drink green juice (two servings a day) and allow ourselves two full meals with snacks. Calorie Limit: 1500.

Weight loss at this stage will be 3 - 3.5 kg. If you feel that you can last longer than four days, feel free to continue this diet for another week. The plumb in this case will be even greater.

Sirtfood Diet: Securing Results

For the period of consolidation is not provided for any strict rules. "Just try to include as many "syrfoods" in your diet as possible in order to feel healthier, more energetic and improve the condition of your skin, as well as becoming even slimmer," says Aidan Goggins.

Keep drinking green juice (one serving a day). General recommendations: dinner should be no later than seven o'clock in the evening, exclude processed foods from the diet, reduce the amount of red meat to 500 g per week. Red wine is allowed and even encouraged, but you can drink it no more than 3 times a week.

This phase can last as long as you need. Many who have appreciated the benefits of sirtfood in their experience prefer to build their entire diet on the basis of sirtfoods.

The Sirrfood Diet Recipes

1. RABBIT WITH APPLES

Energy Value Per Portion

- Calorie Content: 685 Kcal
- Squirrels: 64.3 Gram
- Fats: 37,4 Gram
- Carbohydrates: 21.3 Gram

INGREDIENTS

- Rabbit legs - 4 pieces
- Garlic - 2 cloves
- An Apple - 4 pieces
- Thyme - 4 stems
- Olive oil - 50 ml
- Salt – taste

PREPARATION

1. Crush the cloves of garlic with a knife, add olive oil to them, add thyme and salt, mix all this and marinate the rabbit legs for about an hour.
2. Put the pickled rabbit in a deep form and put in the oven, preheated to 180 degrees, for forty minutes.

3. When this time is up, send the apples cut into large slices into the same form. Bake another fifteen minutes.
4. Serve rabbit legs with baked apples or boiled rice.

2. HUNGARIAN APPLE PIE

ENERGY VALUE PER PORTION

- Calorie Content: 785 Kcal
- Squirrels: 8.7 Gram
- Fats: 27 Gram
- Carbohydrates: 126.9 Gram

INGREDIENTS

- Wheat flour - 130 g
- Sugar - 150 g
- Semolina - 160 g
- Baking powder - 7 g
- Cinnamon - ½ teaspoon
- Butter - 120 g
- An Apple - 7 pieces

PREPARATION

1. Mix flour, semolina, sugar, baking powder and cinnamon in a separate bowl.

2. Wash apples, peel and seed boxes and rub on a coarse grater.
3. We bake the baking dish with baking paper or foil and generously grease with butter.
4. Pour a part of the dry mixture to the bottom of the mold - the layer should not be too thick, and even out. Then we spread the grated apples - with a layer of about the same thickness, level them. Alternating layers spread the whole dry mixture and apples, the last should be a dry layer. I got three dry and two apple layers. Grate the butter on top.
5. Preheat the oven to 180 degrees. Bake the cake for 40–45 minutes - the crust should become rosy.

3. SIMILY SISTERS APPLE PIE

ENERGY VALUE PER PORTION

- Calorie Content: 220 Kcal
- Squirrels: 4,5 Gram
- Fats: 7 Gram
- Carbohydrates: 34.1 Gram

INGREDIENTS

- Yellow apples - 1 kg
- Wheat flour - 150 g
- Sugar - 120 g
- Milk - 100 ml
- Chicken egg - 3 pieces
- Lemon - 1 piece
- Baking powder - 1 teaspoon
- Salt – pinch
- Butter - 50 g
- Cinnamon – taste

PREPARATION

1. Peel and finely chop apples into slices, pour over lemon juice so that they do not darken (sisters recommend the Golden variety).

2. Beat eggs with sugar, salt, zest; add flour with baking powder and milk. Beat everything until smooth.
3. Grease a baking sheet using butter and sprinkle with sugar (a little).
4. Mix 2/3 of the apples with the dough, and randomly put the remaining third on a baking sheet from above (preferably in a round shape 27–28 cm in size). Do not be alarmed - the dough seems very small, but there are a lot of apples. It kind of slightly envelops apples, and that's the point. In the oven, it rises.
5. Take solid butter and put in tiny pieces on apples, sprinkle on top with sugar and cinnamon to taste.
6. Preheat the oven to 180 degrees and bake for 35–40 minutes.
7. You can leave a few slices to put them nicely on top of the cake.

4. WULFS APPLE PIE

ENERGY VALUE PER PORTION

- Calorie Content: 676 Kcal
- Squirrels: 10,4 Gram

- Fats: 41 Gram
- Carbohydrates: 65,4 Gram

INGREDIENTS

- Puff pastry - 500 g
- Sour cream 20% - 400 g
- Honey - 100 g
- Chicken egg - 2 pieces
- An Apple - 5 items
- Butter - 50 g
- Cinnamon – taste

PREPARATION

1. Roll out the puff pastry; put it in a baking sheet. Fry the apples in butter until soft, add honey, cinnamon, mix and remove from heat.
2. Lightly beat the sour cream with two eggs and mix with apples. Put apples and sour cream on rolled dough; wrap the edges of the dough. Lubricate with the remaining beaten egg and place for thirty to forty minutes in the oven, heated to 200 degrees.

5. ALSATIAN APPLE PIE

INGREDIENTS

- Butter - 120 g
- Wheat flour - 180 g
- Salt - ⅓ teaspoon
- Egg yolk - 2 pieces
- Lingonberry - 50 g
- An Apple - 4 pieces
- Chicken egg - 2 pieces
- Sugar - 120 g
- Milk - 150 ml
- Lemon juice - 2 tablespoons

PREPARATION

1. Prepare the dough. To do this, mix the butter with sugar, add 2 yolks, salt and flour.
2. Knead the dough. Form a lump and cool it for 10-15 minutes.
3. Mash the chilled dough in a baking dish greased with oil or lined with parchment baking paper. Pierce with a fork.
4. Bake for 15 minutes in the oven.
5. The filling is done as follows: peel the apples and cut into slices. To prevent apples from darkening, pour them with lemon juice.
6. Fry the apples in a small amount of oil until golden brown.

7. Put the apples in a rose and sprinkle with frozen lingonberries on top, although other berries, such as black currants, are also suitable.
8. For the sauce, mix 2 eggs, 4 tablespoons of sugar and milk.
9. Pour the pie mixture with the mixture.
10. Bake in the oven for 30 minutes.

6. SEMOLINA APPLE PIE

INGREDIENTS

- Wheat flour - 1 cup
- Sugar - 1 cup
- Semolina - 1 cup
- Butter - 50 g
- Soda - 1 teaspoon
- An Apple - 1,5 kg

PREPARATION

1. Mix flour, sugar, semolina and soda.
2. Wash apples, peel and rub on a fine grater.
3. Lubricate the deep form with oil.
4. And the fun begins! We spread the resulting mixture in layers: 1 layer - a dry mixture, 2 layers - grated apples, etc. (I get about 3 apple layers and, accordingly, 4 from dry ingredients), the last layer should be from flour, sugar and semolina!
5. We equate everything, rub on top with frozen (!) Oil (sometimes use margarine for baking Pyshechka).
6. Put in the oven for about 1 hour at 150-200 degrees.

7. Check the readiness with a toothpick; it is necessary that the cake is not wet!
8. We get it, turn it into a dish and wait for it to cool completely.

7. PROVENCAL APPLE PIE WITH WALNUTS

Energy Value Per Portion

- Calorie Content: 310 Kcal
- Squirrels: 6.8 Gram
- Fats: 6.4 Gram
- Carbohydrates: 55 Gram

INGREDIENTS

- Egg white - 2 pieces
- Cane sugar - ½ cup
- Vanilla extract - 1 teaspoon
- Baking powder - 1 teaspoon
- Ground cinnamon - ½ teaspoon
- Wheat flour - ½ cup
- Walnuts - 35 g
- An Apple - 2 pieces

PREPARATION

1. Peel the apples, cut it into half and remove the core. Cut into small cubes.

2. Preheat the oven to 180 degrees. Butter a small baking pan or pan.
3. In a bowl, beat the whites, vanilla, sugar, baking powder and cinnamon. Then add flour, nuts and apples. Mix well.
4. Transfer the dough into the prepared form and bake for 30 minutes until cooked.

8. WARSAW APPLE PIE

INGREDIENTS

- An Apple - 7 pieces
- Wheat flour - 1 cup
- Semolina - 1 cup
- Sugar - 1 cup
- Butter - 100 g
- Lemon - 1 piece
- Cinnamon – taste
- Orange zest – taste

PREPARATION

1. To prepare the filling, wash the apples, peel and grate on a coarse grater. Pour the apples with lemon juice so that they do not darken. Sprinkle

apples with cinnamon, you can also add orange zest.
2. Take a round baking dish and line it with baking paper. If you do not have paper, you can oil the mold. But keep in mind that the Warsaw pie is crumbly, so if you bake it without paper, then it will be difficult to get it out of shape. Combine the flour, semolina, sugar and baking powder and pour a third of the flour mixture into the bottom of the mold. After leveling, lay on top a third of the apples. Alternate layers of apples and dry mix. Lay slices of margarine or butter on the last layer.
3. Bake the Warsaw pie in the oven, heated to 180-200 degrees, for 30-40 minutes (a crust should appear on the pie). Remove the cake from the oven, cool and transfer to a dish - and Warsaw apple pie can be served.

9. SIMPLE APPLE PIE

Energy Value Per Portion

- Calorie Content: 488 Kcal
- Squirrels: 10.7 Gram
- Fats: 5.9 Gram
- Carbohydrates: 97.5 Gram

INGREDIENTS

- Sugar - 1 cup
- Chicken egg - 3 pieces
- Wheat flour - 1 cup
- An Apple - 2 pieces
- Baking powder - ½ teaspoon

PREPARATION

1. Break three eggs into a bowl, add sugar and beat with a mixer until white foam.
2. Then add flour and baking powder, and mix everything.
3. Cut the apples into slices, remove the core.
4. Grease a baking dish with butter, sprinkle with breadcrumbs and lay apples on the bottom. Pour dough and bake for about 40 minutes at medium temperature. The readiness of the pie can then be

checked with a toothpick or a match - the pie is ready when the dough does not stick to the toothpick when it is immersed deep into the pie.

10. Sand Cheese And Apple Pie

INGREDIENTS

- Cinnamon – pinch
- Cottage cheese - 500 g
- An Apple - 1 kg
- Baking powder - 1 teaspoon
- Margarine - 200 g
- Sugar - 1.5 cups
- Wheat flour - 2 cups
- Sour cream - 100 g
- Chicken egg - 4 pieces

PREPARATION

1. For the test, grind 3 yolks (we carefully separate them with proteins) with 0.5 cups of sugar, then grind with softened (not melted) margarine (butter), then introduce the flour, baking powder, knead a rather thick dough with your hands, finally mix in roll sour cream into a bowl, cover and refrigerate for at least half an hour while the filling is being prepared and the oven is preheated
2. Rub the cottage cheese, mix with 1/3 cup sugar and 1 yolk (add the protein from the egg to the remaining three)

3. Peel the apples and seeds, cut into thin slices (until the dough is rolled out, it is better to sprinkle them with lemon juice or diluted citric acid so that they do not darken, but you can cut them already when the cake is ready to be planted in the oven).
4. Roll out the dough thin enough on a rather large baking sheet, making sides along the edges (so that the curd does not drip). We spread evenly the curd filling, beautifully lay the apple slices on it, and sprinkle with cinnamon. We put the oven preheated to 200 degrees for 30-40 minutes.
5. While the cake is baking, beat the whites with the remaining sugar in a thick foam.
6. Take out the slightly baked cake and lay the protein foam over the apples evenly, level it and put it in the hot oven again. When in a few minutes the squirrels grab a light brown crust - the cake is ready!!!

11. DORADO WITH CITRUS PESTO SAUCE

INGREDIENTS

- 2 servings
- 2 pcs Dorado (whole)
- 20 gr Basil

- 1.5 tbsp. l Pine nuts
- 1/4 pcs Lemon (juice and zest)
- 40 ml Olive oil (plus fish oil)
- 1 tbsp. l Parmesan (grated)
- Rosemary / thyme / garlic optional

PREPARATION

1. To clean the fish, remove the gills and make deep cruciform incisions on each side. Season and grease with olive oil (I put it inside on a sprig of thyme and rosemary and a clove of garlic). Bake for 20-30 minutes inside the oven or cook on the barbecue.
2. Cook the pesto. To do this, punch basil in a blender (leave a few leaves for decoration), pine nuts, parmesan, lemon juice and lemon peel and olive oil fried in a dry pan. Add another clove of garlic.
3. Serve the fish with pesto sauce and garnish with basil leaves

12. CITRUS JAM

INGREDIENTS

- 1.5 kg Mandarin
- 5-6 pcs. Oranges
- 1 kg. Sugar
- 1 stick Cinnamon
- 2 tbsp. Pectin
- 2 tbsp. Sahara

PREPARATION

1. Peel tangerines, oranges. I added 1/4 orange zest.
2. Pour sugar overnight. In the morning
3. Mix everything and put it to boil, add cinnamon during the cooking process.
4. After about 30 minutes of cooking, mix the pectin with sugar and pour into the jam
5. Mix well and boil for another 1 minute.
6. Remove from heat, cool, pour into banks.

13. CITRUS CURD CASSEROLE

INGREDIENTS

- 500 grams cottage cheese

- 100g natural yogurt
- 2 pcs the eggs
- 100g rice flour
- Orange zest
- 10 grams vanilla or vanilla sugar
- Taste Sugar

PREPARATION

1. Beat cottage cheese, yogurt and eggs with a blender. Grate the orange peel on a fine grater. Add the zest to the resulting mixture and mix.
2. Add flour, sugar and vanilla to the finished mixture. Preheat the oven to 180 *. Bake until cooked for 30-40 minutes.

14.BLUEBERRY CITRUS SMOOTHIE

INGREDIENTS

- Banana - 2 pcs.

- Orange juice - 2 tbsp.
- Sugar demerara from the mistral - 1 tablespoon
- Blueberries - 2/3 tbsp.
- Ginger - a pinch

PREPARATION

1. Break a banana into pieces.
2. Add blueberries.
3. Add orange juice and a pinch of ginger to the blender bowl.
4. Beat everything in a blender bowl.
5. Pour into glasses, garnish with blueberries or a slice of orange.

15. COCKTAIL OF THREE TYPES OF CITRUS WITH MAPLE SYRUP

INGREDIENTS

- Orange juice - 30 ml.
- Grapefruit juice - 30 ml.
- Lemon juice - 15 ml.
- Maple syrup - 15 ml.
- Ice - 5 cubes
- Highly carbonated mineral water - 50 ml.

-

PREPARATION

1. Squeeze juice from orange, grapefruit, lemon.
2. Measure the required amount and pour into a shaker.
3. Send there the maple syrup and 5 ice cubes. Beat.
4. Pour the contents of the shaker right into a glass, add mineral water and 2 ice cubes and serve!

16. QUINOA, SHRIMP AND CITRUS SALAD

INGREDIENTS

- Salad leaves - 50-70 gr.
- Mistral Quinoa - 1 Cup
- Peeled shrimps (large) - 100 gr.
- Citrus mix (filet grape + sweet) - 150 gr.
- Parmesan (chopped) - 50 gr.
- Salt
- Pepper
- Sweet red pepper
- Vegetable oil for frying
- Olive oil

PREPARATION

1. Make KINOA groats according to the directions on the packaging.
2. Slightly fry the shrimps in vegetable oil, salt a little, sprinkle with sweet red pepper.

Prepare salad dressing:

3. Mix in equal amounts (3-4 tablespoons) olive oil and citrus juice.
4. Salt, pepper, to taste.
5. Dress the resulting quinoa cereal with the resulting sauce.
6. Add the parmesan and lettuce leaves.
7. Put the mixture in a salad bowl with shrimp and citrus slices.

17. CITRUS MIX PUDDING

INGREDIENTS

- Citruses - 3 pcs. (Sweet + grape + orange)
- Eggs - 2 pcs. (s)
- Corn starch - 2 tbsp.
- Cane sugar
- Unrefined demerara from the mistral - 3 tbsp. +4 tsp
- Baked milk - 350 ml.

- Wheat bread - 150-170 g.

PREPARATION

1. Prepare citrus fruits: wash the fruits, cut the peel with a sharp knife, cut the fillet between the separation membranes, cut the citrus pulp into pieces.
2. Beat eggs with 3 tbsp. of cane sugar, add starch, mix, stir constantly, and pour in cold milk.
3. Prepare pudding molds (4 200 ml refractory cups.)
4. Turn on the oven 180 degrees. Put the water to heat up (~ 1.5 liters)
5. Bread (yesterday's and further ... baking) cut into a dice, or cut into the shape of a glass (you need two "circles" per glass).
6. Place the bread disks in the milk mixture; let them "get wet" well.
7. At the bottom of the glass, put the bread circle, then 1 tbsp. of citrus pulp, pour 2 tbsp. milk mixture (mix, as starch has the ability to "settle"), then repeat - bread + citruses + pour the remaining milk. Top with a teaspoon of cane sugar in each glass.
8. Place glasses with puddings in a baking dish; pour hot water into the pan between the glasses (half the pan).

9. Cook the puddings for about 30 minutes. During cooking, the top of the pudding rises, the sugar is caramelized.

Serve puddings in any form. Or immediately after cooking, or let them cool and put in the refrigerator.

18. CARROT SALAD WITH CITRUS MARINADE WITH CHANAH CHEESE

INGREDIENTS

- Carrots - 3 pcs.
- Orange - 1 pc.
- Lime - 1 pc.
- Sugar - 3 tablespoons
- Chanakh cheese - 100 g
- Cilantro - 3 branches
- Chili pepper - 1/4 pc.
- Pine nuts - a handful
- Vegetable oil for deep fat - 1
- Pea seedlings for decoration
- Salt, freshly ground pepper

PREPARATION

1. Wash the carrots, chop with thin cubes;
2. Pour vegetable oil to the bowl of the multicooker no more than up to the "1" mark, that is, no more than 1 liter, close the lid and turn on the FRYTUR program, short mode;
3. When the oil is heated to the temperature necessary for frying, the countdown will begin,

open the lid, insert the basket, put the carrots in it, and fry with the lid open;
4. Cooking hot marinade. Squeeze the orange juice and remove the zest from it, combine in a small saucepan the juice and orange zest, half lime juice with 3 tbsp. sugar, add finely chopped chili, freed from seeds. Boil the syrup;
5. Carrots removed from the deep fryer, first spread on paper napkins to get rid of excess oil, then transfer to a bowl, fill with marinade and leave to stand for 10-15 minutes. Add cilantro leaves to the carrots;
6. Cheese chanah (can be replaced with feta or feta cheese) cut into small cubes;
7. Put carrots in a marinade with cilantro on a dish, slices of cheese, sprinkle with a handful of pine nuts, slightly fried in a dry pan, add salt to taste, garnish with pea seedlings. Season with freshly ground black pepper.

19. ORANGE CITRUS AND PERSIMMON SALAD

INGREDIENTS

- 1 grapefruit
- 1 orange

- 1 persimmon
- 2 tbsp. l acidophilus
- 1 tbsp. l balsamic sauce
- A pinch of orange pepper

PREPARATION

1. With peeling grapefruit and orange.
2. Cut segments out of grapefruit.
3. Cut the orange into thin slices.
4. Cut persimmons into eights.
5. Put orange slices on a beautiful plate, then grapefruit segments and in the center of the persimmon wedges.
6. Sprinkle the whole composition with a pinch of orange pepper.
7. For the sauce, mix acidophilus and balsamic sauce.
8. Then you can pour fruit sauce, or you can just dip fruit slices in the sauce and enjoy.
9. If desired, you can pour fruit with honey or sprinkle with brown sugar.

20. MANNIK COTTAGE CHEESE "STRAWBERRIES WITH CREAM"

INGREDIENTS

- Fat cottage cheese-800 gr.
- Semolina-5 tbsp.
- Eggs - 3-4 pcs.
- Salt-1/2 tsp
- Sugar 1/2 tbsp. (adjust to your liking)
- Vanilla
- Dried fruits (raisins or whatever you like. a citrus flavor, candied pamello)

For cream and filling:

- Fresh strawberries_200-300 gr.
- Fat cream (sour cream) -3-4 tablespoons
- Sugar.

PREPARATION

1. Wipe the cottage cheese through a fine sieve.
2. Blatter the eggs with sugar, salt and vanilla, add the egg mixture to the curd, put the semolina, sliced candied fruit, mix and put into the mold, pre-greased it with vegetable oil and sprinkled with cereal.

3. Cut the strawberries into plates; lay them tightly on the curd dough.
4. Separately, prepare the cream, whip the sour cream or cream with sugar and apply the cream on the strawberries.
5. Bake the manna until cooked, but do not overdo it in the oven.

21. PUMPKIN CITRUS DESSERT

INGREDIENTS

- Pumpkin - 300 g
- Apple - 1 pc
- Orange - 2 pcs
- Honey - 1 tbsp.
- Cinnamon
- Vanillin

PREPARATION

1. Dice Pumpkin
2. Peel the apple and also cut into cubes
3. Remove the zest from the oranges and squeeze the juice
4. Put pumpkin, apple, and zest in a saucepan, pour orange juice, add honey, cinnamon and vanillin to taste.

5. Put on fire and simmer under the lid for about 7-10 minutes.
6. Then turn it off and leave to cool.
7. When it cools down, mashed with a blender, put in a bowl and put in the refrigerator.
8. Let it brew (it took me a whole night), garnish with nuts, cream, or, as I had, a spoon of muesli.

22."LEMONADE" FROM.... CUCUMBERS

INGREDIENTS

- 2 medium cucumbers
- 2 tbsp. lemon juice (can be replaced with any citrus)
- 2 tbsp. honey (can be replaced with sugar, but honey is healthier)
- 100-150 gr. water (boiled, non-carbonated, sparkling, purified, etc.)

PREPARATION

1. Peel the cucumbers as thin as possible, cut into small rings.
2. Put cucumbers, lemon juice, honey and water in a blender and beat for five minutes until airy.
3. You can add ice to the heat. Chill out!

23. PINEAPPLE - CITRUS SORBET WITH LIQUOR

INGREDIENTS

- Pineapple - 1 pc. Weighing approximately 6oo gr.
- Brown sugar - 40 gr.
- Lemon - 1 pc.
- Orange - 1 pc.
- Egg whites - 3 pcs.
- Water - 2 tbsp.
- Liqueur "maraschino" or any other - 10 ml.

PREPARATION

1. Pineapple peels and cut lengthwise into 4 parts. Remove the hard middle.
2. Cut into small pieces and grind in a blender until the consistency of mashed potatoes.
3. Wash the lemon and orange and remove only the top layer of the skin, cut into thin strips. Set aside.
4. Squeeze juice out of lemon and orange.
5. Mix water with sugar and heat over medium heat until the sugar is completely dissolved.
6. Add the citrus juice and boil for another 5 minutes, so that the liquid evaporates a little. Let it cool slightly.

7. Mix the resulting syrup with mashed potatoes, add liquor, and mix thoroughly.
8. Close the container with a lid or cling film and place in the freezer for 2 hours.
9. Remove and mix well until cream.
10. Cover and put in the freezer again for 1 hour.
11. Beat the squirrels in stable foam; gradually mix into a chilled mass.
12. Return to the freezer.
13. For 1 hour before use, get it; let it thaw a little, in order to get the consistency of melted ice cream.
14. Put in portioned bowls, garnish with strips of citrus or at your own discretion.

24. MULLED WINE

Energy Value Per Portion

- Calorie Content: 290 Kcal
- Squirrels: 0.9 Gram
- Fats: 0.4 Gram
- Carbohydrates: 43 Gram

Ingredients

- Sugar - 200 g
- An Apple - 2 pieces

- Oranges - 1 piece
- Cinnamon – pinch
- Nutmeg – pinch
- Clove - 1 piece
- Dry red wine - 1 liter

PREPARATION

1. Bring a mixture of wine, sugar, diced apples, sliced oranges and spices to a boil, remove from heat, and leave for 10 minutes. Then strain and pour into glasses.

25. CHRISTMAS MULLED WINE

INGREDIENTS

- Dry red wine - ¾ l
- Water - ¾ l
- An Apple - 2 pieces
- Oranges - 2 pieces
- Honey - 200 g
- Cinnamon – taste
- Clove – taste
- Anise (star anise) – taste
- Cardamom – taste

- Nutmeg – taste
- Ginger – taste
- Karkade - 1 tablespoon
- Black tea - 1 tablespoon

PREPARATION

1. Pour water inside a pan and bring to a boil.
2. Pour tea and spices. Use must not be ground spices; otherwise the mulled wine will turn cloudy.
3. Pour wine, add chopped fruits and honey.
4. Without taking it to a boil, remove from heat.
5. Serve hot with gingerbread.

26. NON-ALCOHOLIC MULLED WINE

INGREDIENTS

- Grape juice - 3 cups
- Water - ½ cup
- Orange zest - 2 tablespoons
- Lemon zest - 2 tablespoons
- An Apple - ½ pieces
- Raisins - 2 tablespoons
- Cinnamon - 1 teaspoon
- Clove - ½ teaspoon
- Cardamom – pinch
- Ginger - 1 g

PREPARATION

1. Pour grape juice into the pan, add water and fill in all the other ingredients.

2. Put the pan on low heat, not boiling.

3. Allow the mulled wine to brew for 5 minutes under the lid and pour it into the glasses.

27. MULLED WINE WITH COFFEE AND COGNAC

Energy Value Per Portion

- Calorie Content: 245 Kcal
- Squirrels: 0.3 Gram
- Fats: 0 Gram
- Carbohydrates: 25,4 Gram

Ingredients

- Dry red wine - 750 ml
- Espresso - 1.5 cups
- Cognac - ¾ cup
- Sugar - 150 g

PREPARATION

1. Mix wine, coffee (espresso or just strong without thickening), brandy or brandy, sugar and put on moderate heat.

2. Stir until the sugar till it's dissolved, bring the mixture to a boil and immediately remove from heat.

3. Serve hot in mugs or refractory glasses.

28. FRUIT MULLED WINE

Energy Value Per Portion

- Calorie Content: 1297 Kcal
- Squirrels: 1.3 Gram

- Fats: 0.5 Gram
- Carbohydrates: 148.9 Gram

Ingredients

- Wine in bags - 10
- Oranges - 1 kg
- An Apple - 1 kg
- Ground cinnamon – taste
- Ground cloves – taste
- Lemon2 pieces
- Honey – taste

PREPARATION

1. Cut the fruit into slices; place all the ingredients in a saucepan.
2. Bring to a boil, crush the fruit a little, remove from heat and let it brew.

29. CHRISTMAS MULLED WINE WITH WHITE WINE AND ORANGES

Energy Value Per Portion

- Calorie Content: 164 Kcal
- Squirrels: 0.5 Gram
- Fats: 0.2 Gram
- Carbohydrates: 20.6 Gram

Ingredients

- Dry white wine - 750 ml
- Sugar - 100 g
- Water - ½ cup
- Cinnamon sticks - 1 piece
- Clove - 3 pieces
- Oranges - 1 piece

Preparation

1. In a small saucepan, mix water with spices and sugar, add slices of orange and put on moderate heat.

2. While stirring it, bring the mixture to a boil and strain.

3. Mix the wine with the cooked broth and heat over moderate heat, not bringing to a boil.

3. Serve hot in refractory glass mugs.

30. WINTER MULLED WINE

INGREDIENT

- Water - 1.5 cups
- Dry red wine - 1.5 cups
- Cinnamon sticks - 2 pieces
- Clove - 3 pieces
- Grated lemon zest – pinch

- Oranges - 1 piece
- Honey - 6 tablespoons
- Sugar - 2 tablespoons
- Anise (star anise) - 3 pieces
- Ground ginger - on the tip of a knife
- Black tea – taste

PREPARATION

1. Pour water into a pot and bring to a boil.

2. Throw tea and spices.

3. Pour the wine and toss the sliced orange.

4. Add sugar and honey.

5. Cook for 6 minutes without boiling.

31. BUCKWHEAT MEATBALLS WITH MUSHROOMS

INGREDIENTS

- Buckwheat groats - 200 g raw
- Potato - 2 pcs. (large)
- Champignons - 500 g
- Onions - 2 pcs.
- Dill - 20 g
- Vegetable oil - 2 tbsp.

- Ground black pepper and salt - to taste
- Flour for breading - 3-4 tbsp.

PREPARATION

1. Cooking time depends on the preliminary preparation of the ingredients. If you boil potatoes and buckwheat in advance, then it will take you very little time to cook the cutlets themselves.
We will sort and buckwheat. Boil buckwheat at the rate of 1 cup buckwheat in 2 cups of water, pour buckwheat with the boiling water, and add a pinch of salt. We prepare friable porridge, for this we simmer it over medium heat for 15-20 minutes after the water has boiled again. We need all the liquid to evaporate and the cereal to boil.
2. Boil the potatoes in their skins until ready in boiling water for 15-25 minutes. Cooking time depends on size and variety of potatoes. Check the potatoes for readiness with a fork or knife. The knife should easily enter the potato. Cool the finished potatoes, then peel and rub on a medium grater.
3. Onion cut into small cubes.
4. Pour the vegetable oil into the pan, heat it and fry the onions for 7 minutes, until tender, stirring occasionally.
5. Cut the mushrooms into a very small cube.

6. Add mushrooms to the onion, salt and pepper vegetables to taste. Cook the vegetables for another 10 minutes.
7. Now put in a bowl all the ingredients for our lean cutlets: boiled buckwheat, grated potatoes, fried mushrooms with onions, chopped dill. You can add seasoning for vegetables.
8. We shift the minced meat into a blender and punch it well until smooth.
9. We form cutlets of any shape from the resulting stuffing. Bone cutlets either in flour or in breadcrumbs. You can fry lean buckwheat cutlets with mushrooms in a pan with the addition of oil. Cook them in deep fat at 180 degrees 5 minutes. We put ready cutlets on a paper towel to get rid of excess oil.

32. BUCKWHEAT CHICKEN CUTLETS

INGREDIENTS

- Chilled Chicken
- Boiled buckwheat - 200 g
- Onion - 1 head
- Garlic - 3 cloves
- Chicken Egg - 1 pc.
- Salt to taste
- Sunflower oil - for frying
- Bread to taste

PREPARATION

1. Chicken breast and fillet cut from chicken legs are suitable for minced meat. We do not use skin. Twist the breast and fillet in a meat grinder.
2. Twist boiled buckwheat in chicken minced meat.
3. Onions and garlic. Let's break the chicken egg. Add salt.
4. Stir the minced meat into a homogeneous cutlet mass.
5. We form balls of the same size with wet hands. Roll the balls in breading, squeeze gently into the patty. We send the cutlets to a preheated pan. First, pour the sunflower oil into the pan.

6. Fry chicken cutlets with buckwheat on both sides over medium heat. Then close up the pan with a lid and switch to a slow fire. Bring our cutlets to readiness under the lid for 30 minutes.

33. BUCKWHEAT DIET CUTLETS

INGREDIENTS

- Buckwheat groats - 200 g
- Chicken Egg - 1 pc.
- Onion - 1 head
- Salt to taste
- Vegetable oil - for frying
- Breadcrumbs - to taste
- Fresh greens - to serve

PREPARATION

1. Boil buckwheat until fully cooked. In the process of cooking, buckwheat needs to be slightly salted. Buckwheat is cooked for 15-20 minutes, depending on the quality of the cereal. To make buckwheat friable, pour two fingers up on the water. Put the cooled boiled groats in a bowl. If you still have buckwheat porridge from breakfast, then blind the cutlets from it.

2. Onions cut into cubes. Add to buckwheat. Let's break the chicken egg.
3. A little salt does not hurt.
4. Using a submersible blender, mix everything into the buckwheat.
5. Add the breadcrumbs. Stir the minced meat with a spoon, add crackers in small portions until the stuffing becomes thick, with wet hands we will form buckwheat cutlets.
6. Preheat the pan. Add vegetable oil. Lightly brown the patties on one side.
7. Turnover and lightly brown on the other side. Then turn down the heat to a minimum. We put out the buckwheat cutlets under the lid for another 10 minutes. If necessary, add a third of a glass of water to the pan. Buckwheat diet cutlets are ready! Fast, cheap and cheerful.

34. BUCKWHEAT CUTLETS

INGREDIENTS

- Buckwheat (cooked) - 680 g
- Bouillon cube - 1 pc. (10 g);
- Onions - 0.5 pcs.

- Chicken Egg - 1 pc.
- Garlic - 2 cloves
- Breadcrumbs - 6 tbsp.
- Vegetable oil for frying - how much is needed

PREPARATION

1. Cook in advance loose buckwheat porridge, let it cool. Also prepare bouillon cube, onion, egg, garlic, breadcrumbs, and vegetable oil. In crumbly buckwheat porridge, cooked in not too salty water, crumble the bouillon cube.
2. Break the egg in buckwheat, add the onion and garlic (large cubes).
3. In a blender or in a food processor, beat the buckwheat with the rest of the ingredients. All this should turn into a mass, reminiscent of both consistency and appearance of minced meat.
4. Blind cutlets from buckwheat mincemeat (15 pieces) and bread them in breadcrumbs.
5. Fry the buckwheat cutlets in vegetable oil until crusted. Since meatballs are not made from minced meat, they do not need to be fried for a long time or stewed later.

35. BUCKWHEAT AND COTTAGE CHEESE CUTLETS

INGREDIENTS

- Buckwheat groats - 1 cup
- Cottage cheese - 200-250 g
- Greens – optional
- Salt to taste
- Wheat flour - 1-2 tbsp.
- Spices to taste
- Oil - for frying
- Flour - for breading

PREPARATION

1. Prepare buckwheat, cottage cheese, spices and flour.
2. Cook ordinary buckwheat from buckwheat (do not forget to salt it, but you cannot add oil).
3. Add cottage cheese, spices (you can take black pepper, curry, paprika, asafoetida ...), salt and any greens (fresh or dried), if any. Mash all ingredients thoroughly with your hands to get the most homogeneous mass. Add the flour a little to make the mincemeat begin to form well.
4. Form small cutlets, bread them in flour.
5. Fry in vegetable oil on both sides.

6. Serve hot cutlets of buckwheat and cottage cheese.

36. MEATBALLS WITH BUCKWHEAT IN A SLOW COOKER

INGREDIENTS

- Minced meat - 250 g
- Buckwheat - 1/2 cup
- Chicken Egg - 1 pc.
- Onions - 1-2 pcs.
- Carrots - 1 pc.
- Flour - 1 tbsp.
- Sour cream - 2 tablespoons
- Vegetable oil - 1 tbsp.
- Salt, pepper - to taste

PREPARATION

1. Boil buckwheat in advance until half cooked. Finely chop the onion or mince it with minced meat. In the bowl, put the minced meat, buckwheat, onion, add the egg. Salt and pepper to taste.

2. We mix the ingredients, let the minced meat "rest" for several minutes. We form meatballs weighing approximately 40-50 g.
3. In vegetable oil, fry meatballs with buckwheat in a slow cooker on both sides for 10 minutes in the "Frying" mode. Gently turn the meatballs with a plastic or wooden spoon.
4. Put the meatballs on a plate for now, cover with a bowl. We will prepare the sauce.
5. While the meatballs are fried, grate the carrots on a coarse grater, chop the onion finely. Let's send the vegetables to the slow cooker - to the oil remaining from frying. In the "Frying" mode, we spice the vegetables for 10 minutes, stirring.
6. Add flour, mix quickly. Add sour cream to the vegetables and pour water. If you like thick gravy - pour 2 cups of water, if more liquid - 3 cups. You can slightly salt and add spices. Now put the meatballs in the sauce. It is not necessary that they be completely covered with sauce.
7. Put the "Extinguishing" program for 20 minutes. And now our magnificent dish is ready! Delicate meatballs with buckwheat in sour cream sauce served with your favorite side dish or with fresh vegetables.

37. BUCKWHEAT CUTLETS (LEAN)

INGREDIENTS

- Buckwheat - 150 g
- Water - 300 ml
- Onions - 150 g
- Carrots - 150 g
- Sunflower oil - 50 g
- Dill - 0.5 tsp
- Dried basil - 0.5 tsp
- Salt to taste
- Ground black pepper - to taste
- Ground caraway seeds - a pinch
- Breadcrumbs - 30 g

PREPARATION

1. Boil buckwheat until cooked, without salt.
2. In sunflower oil, fry chopped onions and grated carrots until soft.
3. In a bowl of a food processor, simply place boiled buckwheat and fried vegetables. Grind to a puree state. You can grind several times in a meat grinder.

4. Add dried herbs, caraway seeds, salt, and pepper. Mix well. A viscous mass will be obtained from which it is easy to form cutlets.
5. Form cutlets of any size and breadcrumbs.
6. Heat oil in a pan. Sauté the lean buckwheat cutlets over medium heat until rosy. Since they are very fragile, carefully flip them to the other side.
7. Lay on a paper towel. Buckwheat meatballs are ready. Serve immediately

38. MEATBALLS WITH BUCKWHEAT AND MINCED MEAT

INGREDIENTS

- Buckwheat groats - 120 g
- Minced meat - 300 g
- Egg - 1 pc.
- Onions - 40 g
- Sour cream - 2 tablespoons
- Tomato paste - 1 tbsp.
- Sunflower oil - 40 ml
- Wheat flour - 1 tbsp.
- Salt to taste

PREPARATION

1. Boil buckwheat
2. Add minced meat, chopped onions and egg to buckwheat, salt, knead until smooth. Form small meatballs - the size may be what you are used to, make a little more than a walnut. Bread them in flour.
3. In warmed sunflower oil, fry meatballs with buckwheat and minced meat from all sides.
4. Flip to the other side. The sauce can be made right away, or can be prepared separately.
5. Dry the flour inside a dry frying pan until light pink and a nutty flavor appears. Cool slightly and dilute with water.
6. Dry the flour inside a dry frying pan until light pink and a nutty flavor appears. Cool slightly and dilute with water.
7. Stew meatballs in the resulting sauce.

39. BUCKWHEAT AND MINCED MEATBALLS

INGREDIENTS

- Minced meat - 500 g
- Boiled buckwheat - 200 g
- Onion - 1 pc.

- Garlic - 1 clove
- Chicken Egg - 1 pc.
- Flour - 3 tbsp.
- Vegetable oil - 3 tbsp.
- Salt, pepper - to taste

PREPARATION

1. To prepare buckwheat cutlets with minced meat, we will prepare the products according to the list. Minced meat is better to use pork and beef. Buckwheat is better to pre-boil at the rate of 1 cup of cereal in 2.5 cups of water + salt. Cool the finished buckwheat.
2. Put the minced meat and buckwheat in a bowl.
3. Add the grated onion and let the garlic pass through the press.
4. Add the chicken egg, salt and pepper to the minced meat.
5. Mix the ingredients of the minced meat well.
6. From the minced meat we form cutlets of your usual shape.
7. Bread cutlets in flour.
8. Pour vegetable oil inside the pan and heat it. Fry the patties on one side for 4-5 minutes, then turn and fry the second side for 4-5 minutes. After that,

add 2-3 tbsp. water and then cover the pan with a lid. We put out the patties for another 10 minutes.
9. Cutlets with buckwheat and minced meat are ready!

40. VEGETARIAN CUTLETS WITH BUCKWHEAT AND POTATOES

INGREDIENTS

- Buckwheat groats - 1 cup
- Potato - 500 g
- Flour - 4 tbsp.
- Spices to taste
- Salt to taste
- Vegetable oil - 3 tbsp.

PREPARATION

1. Buckwheat should be washed, pour clean water and leave for 2-3 hours. The longer the buckwheat will stand, the more it will be in volume, up to a certain point, of course, but it must be soaked for at least an hour.
2. Now buckwheat can be chopped with a blender, but can be left as is. Add peeled grated peeled potatoes to the swollen buckwheat.
3. Stir, add salt and spices to taste
4. Stir; gradually add flour, stirring each time.
5. As soon as the mass begins to "sculpt" well, form cutlets. Bread them in flour.

6. Fry vegetarian cutlets with buckwheat and potatoes on both sides in a sufficient amount of oil (cutlets do not take oil in the same way as eggplants, but still). Fold the finished patties back into the pan, add some water and steam under the lid for a few more minutes.

41. EGGPLANT WITH WALNUT AND GARLIC

INGREDIENTS

- Eggplant - 2 pcs.
- Walnuts - 0.5 cups
- Garlic - 1-2 cloves
- Dill - 0.25 beams
- Parsley - 0.25 bunches
- Salt to taste
- Sunflower oil - for frying

PREPARATION

1. In eggplant, cut the tails and cut into slices 3-4 mm thick. Fold the eggplant in a bowl, salt and leave for 30 minutes, then pat it dry with napkins.
2. Heat sunflower oil inside a pan and fry the eggplant on both sides.
3. Then lay the eggplants on paper towels to remove excess oil.

4. Cook the filling. Put peeled walnuts, chopped garlic and herbs in a blender bowl. Garlic should be taken to taste, given the size of the cloves. As greens, Do dill and parsley; you can take cilantro if you like.
5. Grind the filling with the "metal knife" nozzle, then salt a little.
6. Put the fried eggplant strips on a plate, 1-2 tsp on the edge of the strip. Nut-garlic filling. Twist the eggplant into rolls.
7. Put eggplant rolls with walnuts and garlic on a plate, decorate with herbs. You can serve a snack to the table.

42. RED BEAN LOBIO

INGREDIENTS

- Red beans - 1-1.5 cups
- Walnuts - 0.5 cups
- Onion - 1 head
- Garlic - 1 clove
- Tomato juice - 0.5-1 cup
- Vegetable oil - 1-2 tbsp.
- Apple cider vinegar - 1 teaspoon
- Fresh (or dry greens) - to taste
- Ground peppers - to taste
- Hot pepper - 1 pod

- Salt - 1 pinch.

PREPARATION

1. Beans must be soaked for a long time, for example, at night or for 5-8 hours.
2. Then fill with fresh water and cook until soft for about 1 hour. For the dish you will need beans without the resulting broth from cooking, although sometimes a little bean broth is added.
3. Chop walnuts and garlic.
4. Chop off the onion and fry a little in vegetable oil, and then add the prepared beans, tomato juice, walnuts and garlic to it.
5. Stir, add the hot pepper pod on top and simmer over low heat for 10-15 minutes.
6. At the very end of cooking, add greens: fresh and / or dry.

43. GEORGIAN EGGPLANT WITH NUTS

INGREDIENTS

- Eggplant - 500 g
- Walnuts - 100 g
- Vinegar - 1/2 tsp
- Suneli hops to taste

- Garlic - 2 cloves
- Parsley - 20 g
- Cilantro - 20 g
- Salt to taste
- Ground black pepper - 1 pinch

PREPARATION

1. Eggplant for this dish is better to take authentic, but not old. Cut them into strips 2 mm thick. Sprinkle eggplant with coarse salt. Leave them in salt for 10-15 minutes. During this time, eggplant will give their bitterness. After that, wash them under running water; dry them with paper towels to get rid of moisture.
2. Prepare a dietary version of the dish, fry eggplant; it will be in a dry grill pan. Firstly, the eggplant is juicy, and secondly, in the process of frying, a beautiful pattern on the eggplant strips is obtained, which will give the dish a beautiful appearance. Fry eggplant on both sides for 3-4 minutes. You can fry eggplant in vegetable oil in a pan, and on charcoal, and on a wire rack.
3. Prepare a nut filling. In a blender bowl, lay out walnuts, cilantro and parsley leaves, and cloves of garlic, suneli hop and water. Punch everything in a blender to a puree state.

4. In the finished walnut puree, add wine vinegar, salt and black pepper.
5. Prepare the fried eggplant and nut filling and proceed to roll the rolls.
6. Spread a teaspoon of nut filling from the wide edge of the strip and gently twist the eggplant into a roll. Do this with all strips of eggplant.

44. COOKIES "CIGARETTES" WITH NUTS

INGREDIENTS

Dough:

- Flour - 460-500 g
- Butter - 200 g
- Sour cream - 200 g
- Salt - 0.3 tsp
- Vanillin - a pinch

Filling:

- Walnuts - 1.5 cups
- Sugar - 1 cup
- Honey - 2-3 tbsp.
- Egg - for lubrication
- Powdered sugar - for sprinkling
- Glass - 250 ml

PREPARATION

1. Sift flour and mix with vanilla and salt. Chop the butter and grind it with your hands with flour until fine crumbs are obtained.
2. In the center, make an hole and add sour cream.
3. Mix the dough with a spoon. Get friable mass, as in the photo. Then, with your hands, collect the

dough in a single lump and mix lightly so as not to delay the process.
4. Place the dough in a film and put in the refrigerator while preparing the filling.
5. Slightly fry the walnuts in a dry pan and grind in a blender until fine crumbs. It is undesirable to grind nuts until a smooth paste.

45. LUXURIOUS COOKIES

INGREDIENTS

- Chicken egg (protein) - 1 pc.
- Powdered Sugar - 50 g
- Walnuts - 50 g
- Coconut Chips - 50 g
- Chocolate - 50 g
- Prunes - 50 g

PREPARATION

1. Beat the egg white with powdered sugar into a white lush mass.
2. Add coconut and chopped chocolate.

3. Also chop coarsely nuts and chop prunes.
4. Mix.
5. Cover the baking sheet. Spoon the mass with small balls of lumps.
6. Put cookies in the oven preheated to 180 degrees and bake for one minute. Disconnect.
7. Do not open the door. As the oven cools completely, you can take out cookies and pour tea.

46. COOKIES "MAZURKA" WITH WALNUTS AND RAISINS

INGREDIENTS

- Raisins - 1 cup
- Walnuts - 1 cup
- Chicken eggs - 2 pcs.
- Wheat flour - 1 cup
- Sugar - 1 cup
- Dough baking powder - 1.5 tsp.
- Butter - 10 g to lubricate the mold

PREPARATION

1. Let's start making cookies by separating the whites from the yolks.

2. In a bowl, beat sugar with proteins with a mixer until stable peaks.
3. Add the yolk to the sugar-protein mass. Mix everything with a mixer.
4. Add the baking powder to the bowl.
5. At the very end, add the flour and knead the dough.
6. If your raisins are too dry, you can pre-soak it in hot water for 15-20 minutes and then drain the water. Add raisins to the dough.
7. Grind walnuts in a mortar.
8. Add the nuts to the bowl to the rest of the dough ingredients. Mix again all the ingredients of the dough
9. A baking dish or a baking sheet with a sheet of parchment paper (grease it with butter) or a silicone mat, spread the dough in a thin layer, up to 1 cm thick, over the sheet and send it to a preheated to 190-200 degrees C for 15 minutes.
10. This is what the Mazurka cookies look like with walnuts and raisins after baking
11. Hot cut the cookies into rhombuses or squares of any size.
12. Let the Mazurka cookies cool and serve.

47. ABKHAZIAN EGGPLANT

INGREDIENTS

- Eggplant - 2 pcs.
- Walnuts - 80 g
- Parsley - 20 g
- Cilantro - 20 g
- Onions - 60 g
- Garlic - 2 cloves
- Suneli hops - 5 g
- Salt to taste
- Wine vinegar - 1 tbsp.
- Vegetable oil for frying - 3 tbsp.

PREPARATION

1. Peel and slice the eggplant in longitudinal slices. Salt on all sides and let lie for about 5 minutes, then rinse with salt and squeeze well.
2. Fry the eggplant plates in a well-heated oil pan. Put on a paper towel so that excess oil is absorbed into the towel.
3. Crush the nuts, Do it with a coffee grinder; try not to turn into flour.
4. Finely chop the onion, add chopped herbs.
5. Add garlic crushed garlic into the mixture.

6. Stir the resulting mixture. Add vinegar (I haven't found any wine, I've taken a balsamic one, and the aroma will be different) and hops-suneli. If too cool, pour in water so that the mass can be slightly smeared.
7. It remains to stuff the plates of eggplant. On one half of the fried strip, spread the nut-spicy filling.
8. We cover with the second half. So do with all the plates of eggplant.
9. We spread the eggplants in Abkhazian style on a dish, let it brew for a few hours, and serve as a snack, garnished with onion rings, herbs, pomegranate seeds.

48.nPUFF PASTRY ROLL WITH APPLES

INGREDIENTS

- Puff pastry - 500 g
- Apples - 700 g
- Walnut - 100 g
- Raisins - 50 g (optional)
- Butter - 40 g
- Cinnamon - 0.5-1 tsp (taste)
- Sugar - 70-100 g (to taste)
- Wheat flour - for working with dough
- Chicken Egg - 1 pc. (optional)
- Powdered sugar - 1 tbsp. (optional)

PREPARATION

1. Peel off the apples, take out the core and cut into four parts. We cut each part into thin slices.
2. Melt a piece of butter in a frying pan, add chopped apples and, stirring occasionally, simmer the apples for 5-7 minutes without covering.
3. Add sugar and ground cinnamon to the apples. Stir, put out still 3 minutes. The amount of sugar should be regulated depending on the sweetness of apples, to your liking. Add 50 grams of sugar

immediately, and when the sugar has melted, try the filling and add more if necessary.
4. Turning off the fire, completely cool the filling before proceeding with further cooking. While the filling is cooling, we will also unfreeze the puff pastry, leaving it at room temperature for 30-40 minutes.
5. Pour raisins with hot water and leave for 5-10 minutes, so that it swells a little.
6. Grind the walnuts with a knife, in a blender or coffee grinder to the state of small crumbs.
7. We lay out the puff pastry on a surface sprinkled with flour and divide into two parts. We remove one part in the refrigerator, and in the meantime we roll out the second to a thickness of about 2-3 mm.
8. Sprinkle the dough with half the crumbs, so that 2-3 cm of clean dough is left along its vertical edges and near horizontal, and about 7-8 cm along the far edge of the dough.
9. Put the chilled apple filling on the nut crumbs.
10. With raisins, salt the water as much as possible (you can squeeze it slightly to remove excess liquid). Separating half the raisins, distribute it on the surface of the apple filling.

11. Roll the dough with the filling into the roll, tucking the edges and gently pinching the seam. If the kitchen is hot also the dough has softened by this time - place the roll in the refrigerator for 15 minutes before starting to bake.
12. On a baking sheet lined with baking paper, lay the roll seam down. On the top surface of the roll we make cuts every 2-3 cm (cut the top layer of dough to the filling). Lubricate the surface of the roll with a beaten egg.
13. Place the roll in the oven preheated to 180 degrees and bake for 30-35 minutes until golden brown. In the meantime, repeat the whole process with the remaining half of the dough and filling.
14. Puff pastry roll with apples is ready. Cut it into portions, sprinkle with powdered sugar and serve

49. STRING BEAN SALAD WITH WALNUTS

INGREDIENTS

- Green beans - 400 g
- Walnut - 3 tablespoons
- Parsley - 0.5 bunch
- Salad onion - 0.5-1 pcs.

- Olive oil - 4 tsp
- Dijon mustard - 1-2 tsp (taste)
- Wine Red / Balsamic Vinegar - 2 tsp
- Honey - 1-2 tsp (taste)
- Salt to taste
- Ground black pepper to taste

PREPARATION

1. Fry the nuts inside a dry frying pan for several minutes until a nutty flavor appears.
2. Steam the string beans to the desired degree of readiness. For frozen thin green beans, as a rule, 5-8 minutes of cooking over medium heat is enough. Beans should remain resilient, slightly crispy, but delicate in taste.
3. Prepare a salad dressing by mixing olive oil, vinegar, honey and mustard.
4. Cut the red onion into quarters or thin half rings, chop the toasted nuts coarsely, and chop the parsley.
5. Place the steamed beans in a salad bowl. Add onions, nuts and parsley.
   To preserve a bright green color, beans can be pre-doused with cold water, but this should be done quickly so that inside the bean pods remain warm.

6. Add dressing to prepared salad ingredients and mix everything carefully.
7. Add salt and then ground black pepper to taste.
8. Bean salad with walnuts is ready. Serve the salad warm up or at room temperature

50. BANANA CRUMBLE

INGREDIENTS

- Butter - 50 g
- Sugar - 2 tbsp.
- Wheat flour - 3 tbsp. (with a slide)
- Walnut Kernels - 30 g
- Banana - 2 pcs.

PREPARATION

1. Combine cold butter with sugar and flour.
2. Stir with a quick motion with a fork (or rub with your hands) until crumbs form.
3. Chop walnuts with a knife into medium pieces and add to the sand mass. Mix
4. Peel and slice the bananas into small pieces.
5. Put the bananas in a suitable shape. For the preparation of crumble, you can take portioned molds or one large one.
6. On top of the bananas, evenly distribute all the chips.
7. Send the dessert form to the oven preheated to 180 degrees. Bake for 20-25 minutes, until golden brown.
8. Delicious banana crumble can be served.

51. BROWNIES WITH MILK AND DARK CHOCOLATE

INGREDIENTS

- Milk chocolate - 100 g
- Dark chocolate - 100 g
- Wheat flour - 1.25 cups
- Butter - 225 g
- Chicken egg - 4 pieces
- Sugar - 2 cups
- Vanillin – taste
- Salt - 1 teaspoon
- Nuts – taste

PREPARATION

1. Break the chocolate to pieces and melt in a water bath with butter so that there are no lumps left.
2. Add a glass of sugar and mix for 30 seconds. Add vanillin. Remove from heat and allow cooling.
3. Beat two eggs with 0.5 cups of sugar until completely dissolved. Gently pour into the chocolate mixture, stirring constantly. If the chocolate mixture is hot, the eggs can be cooked.

4. Beat the remaining 2 eggs with sugar at full capacity for 5 minutes - the mass should increase in volume by 2 times. Stir in the chocolate mass.
5. Sift flour with salt. Stir in the mixture (I whisk lightly with a mixer). Nuts can be added as desired.
6. Preheat the oven to 180 degrees. Cover the baking dish (about 20x20 cm) with parchment paper and grease with butter or vegetable oil (do not cover paper with disposable forms). It can also be made in the form of cupcakes.
7. Pour the dough (by consistency, it should turn out as a thick sour cream). Level the top and put in the oven on the middle shelf.
8. The baking time depends on the oven for about 25-50 minutes. Readiness is checked with a stick or a knife - if there is liquid chocolate on the tip, and then sends it back to the oven, if there is slightly wet dough, and then the brownie is ready. If baked in the form of cupcakes, then the baking time will be reduced depending on their size. Large, bake for 35 minutes. Serve with various creams or syrups.

52. BROWNIE WITH BANANA AND DARK CHOCOLATE

INGREDIENTS

- Butter - 100 g
- Dark chocolate - 100 g
- Wheat flour - 70 g
- Bananas - 1 piece
- Chicken egg - 2 pieces
- Sugar - 2 tablespoons
- Baking powder - 1 teaspoon

PREPARATION

1. Melt butter and chocolate over low heat. Remove and cool.

2. Beat eggs and sugar with a whisk.

3. Pour chocolate into the sugar mixture. Mix.

4. Pour flour and baking powder. Stir again.

5. Pour the mixture into a baking dish. Cut the banana into thin slices and drown in chocolate.

6. Bake for 30–35 minutes at a temperature of 180 degrees.

7. Cool. Cut into slices, garnish with icing sugar.

53. VANILLA BROWNIE WITH WALNUTS AND DARK CHOCOLATE

INGREDIENTS

- Dark chocolate - 200 g
- Butter - 150 g
- Vanilla extract - 1 teaspoon
- Chicken egg - 4 pieces
- Wheat flour - 100 g
- Cocoa powder - 1.5 tablespoons
- Peeled walnuts - 100 g
- Sugar - ½ cup

PREPARATION

1. Preheat the oven to 180 degrees.

2. Cut the chocolate and butter into pieces and melt together in a water bath. Let cool.

3. Pour sugar into melted chocolate. Add vanilla and eggs, mixing after each.

4. Sift the flour and cocoa; add it to the same mixture.

5. Add nuts here. Pour into the form and bake for 20-25 minutes.

54. BROWNIES WITH WALNUTS AND DARK CHOCOLATE

INGREDIENTS

- Baking powder - 2 teaspoons
- Dark chocolate - 400 g
- Butter - 400 g
- Sugar - 500 g
- Chicken egg - 6 items
- Wheat flour - 250 g
- Walnuts - 300 g

PREPARATION

1. Break the chocolate (300 grams) into pieces, put in a bowl and place in a water bath. Add the diced butter to the chocolate. Melt chocolate with butter until smooth, stirring.
2. Add sugar, mix well and remove the pan from the water bath. If the sugar mixture is quite hot, you need to cool it a bit before introducing the eggs so that the eggs do not curl. Insert eggs one at a time, stirring each time until smooth.
3. Sift flour with baking powder. Pour flour with baking powder into the chocolate-egg mixture and mix.
4. Chop the chocolate (100 grams) and nuts, add to the dough and mix.
5. Lubricate the baking dish with oil, cover with parchment and grease again with a thin layer of oil. Put the dough in the form and flatten.

6. Bake the brownies in an oven heated to 170 degrees for about 35–40 minutes, or until the toothpick comes out dry. The main thing is not to dry the brownie. The cake should remain a little wet. Remove the cake out from the oven and cool, or even better, put it in the refrigerator for 8-12 hours (or overnight).
7. Cut the brownies into square cakes and serve with tea.

55. HOT CHOCOLATE WITH VANILLA AND DARK CHOCOLATE

INGREDIENTS

- Sugar - 4 cups
- Vanilla pod - ½ pieces
- Dark chocolate - 680 g
- Milk chocolate - 230 g
- Cocoa powder - 2 cups
- Milk - 280 ml

PREPARATION

1. Pour sugar into a saucepan and add the vanilla bean, broken in half. Remove the seeds, mash them slightly with your hands and add there. Stir, cover with foil and then leave overnight at room temperature.
2. In a combine, grind both chocolates into crumbs.
3. Remove the vanilla pod from the sugar. Add chocolate and cocoa powder to the sugar. Mix well.
4. For 1 serving, heat 280 ml of milk and add 0.25 cups of the mixture. Mix well. Serve warm, garnished with unsweetened whipped cream.

56. DARK CHOCOLATE CURD CAKE

INGREDIENTS

- Salt – taste
- Wheat flour - 800 g
- Dry yeast - 7 g
- Sugar - 110 g
- Butter - 105 g
- Milk - 175 ml
- Cottage cheese - 225 g
- Dark chocolate - 125 g
- Chicken egg - 3 pieces

PREPARATION

1. Stir the yeast with salt, 150 grams of flour and 100 grams of sugar. Heat milk with 75 grams of butter and 60 ml of water. Beat the cream and milk mixture and combine with the yeast. Mix. Beat 2 eggs and add the remaining flour in portions.
2. Knead the ball from the dough and leave for 1 hour in a warm place.
3. Separate the yolk from the protein. Cool the protein, and beat the yolk with cottage cheese and grated chocolate.
4. Heat the oven to 170 degrees.

5. Knead the dough on a powdery surface and leave for 15 minutes.
6. Transfer the dough to a greased baking sheet and roll into a layer. Put the curd and chocolate filling in the center, roll the edges slightly. Leave on for 30 minutes.
7. Beat the protein with water and grease the cake. Bake for about 50 minutes. If the cake starts to burn, cover with foil.

57. DARK CHOCOLATE BROWNIE IN A PAN

INGREDIENTS

- Butter - 200 g
- Dark chocolate - 100 g
- Milk chocolate - 100 g
- Chicken egg - 4 pieces
- Sugar - 140 g
- Wheat flour - 150 g

PREPARATION

1. Preheat the oven to 180 degrees.

2. In a water bath, melt the butter and two packets of chocolate.

3. Mix eggs with sugar.

4. Add a mixture of chocolate and butter; pour flour into the same place.

5. Grease a frying pan with butter, sprinkle with flour.

6. Pour in the mass.

7. Bake for 30 minutes.

58. SEMOLINA PORRIDGE WITH WHITE AND DARK CHOCOLATE AND DRIED CHERRY

INGREDIENTS

- Milk - 280 ml
- Semolina - 80 g
- White chocolate - 50 g
- Dark chocolate - 30 g
- Almond flakes - 10 g
- Dried cherry - 30 g

PREPARATION

1. Pour milk into a small saucepan. Break the white chocolate and throw into milk. Put the stew pan on medium heat and bring the milk to a boil. When it boils, vigorously whisk the melted chocolate and milk into a homogeneous liquid with a whisk (from this step

onwards, continue to cook the porridge with constant stirring). In a thin stream enter semolina, reduce heat slightly and cook for about 5–6 minutes until thick. Remove the stew pan from the heat, mix the dried cherry and almond flakes into the porridge and immediately pour it onto a warm plate.

2. Break the dark chocolate with your hands, put everything in a heat-resistant plate and put in the microwave for half a minute – minute, periodically opening the door and stirring. Carefully remove the plate, scoop the melted chocolate with a tablespoon and decorate the white surface of the porridge with chocolate bar. Or don't bother and take high-quality dark chocolate chips, pour over the porridge and serve immediately.

59. STRAWBERRY IN DARK CHOCOLATE WITH WHITE PATTERNS

Energy Value Per Portion

- Calorie Content: 735 Kcal
- Squirrels: 7.3 Gram
- Fats: 47.5 Gram
- Carbohydrates: 68,4 Gram

Ingredients

- Dark chocolate - 350 g
- Butter - 1 tablespoon
- Strawberry - 150 g
- White chocolate - 150 g

PREPARATION

1. Cover the pan with parchment.

2. In a bowl, mix the crushed dark chocolate and butter. Put a water bath and melt, stirring, until smooth.

3. Meanwhile, rinse the strawberries well and dry (it is very important that the berries are dry).

4. Holding the ponytails, dip the berries in chocolate and spread on a baking sheet. Leave to harden.

5. Meanwhile, melt the crushed white chocolate in a water bath. Sprinkle strawberries with white chocolate to make zigzag patterns. Leave to solidify.

60. CLASSIC BROWNIE WITH DARK CHOCOLATE AND NUTS

INGREDIENTS

- Dark chocolate - 300 g
- Butter - 200 g
- Wheat flour - 150 g

- Natural coffee - 1 tablespoon
- Chicken egg - 5 items
- Sugar - 230 g
- Vanilla sugar - 1 teaspoon
- Walnuts - 150 g

PREPARATION

1. In a deep container, break the chocolate finely, divide the butter into pieces and melt together in the microwave at low power, periodically checking and mixing the mixture.

2. While the butter and chocolate are mixed, chop nuts, grind coffee and sift it together with flour.

3. In a mixer, beat eggs with sugar and vanilla into a lightened, increased in volume, fluffy mass.

4. In parts, mix the sugar-egg mixture into the chocolate-butter mixture.

5. Add flour, nuts, mix thoroughly.

6. Put the dough in the mold and put the bake in the oven preheated to 180 degrees for 30 minutes.

7. After baking, remove the brownie from the mold, allow to cool and then cut into square pieces. Before serving, ideally heat in the oven or microwave and add ice cream.

61. LAZY PARSLEY AND PARMESAN SALAD

INGREDIENTS

- 2 cloves of garlic
- 6 tbsp. olive oil
- 1 tbsp. lemon juice
- 4 large bunches of young parsley (leaves only)
- 40-50 g of grated hard seasoned cheese on a fine grater, better than parmesan
- Salt, freshly ground black pepper

PREPARATION

1. Use a blender to mix peeled and crushed garlic with olive oil until smooth. Add lemon juice, add salt and pepper and mix well.
2. Before serving, mix finely chopped parsley leaves with grated cheese in a bowl and pours the dressing over it.

NOTE: Instead of parsley, the basis of such a salad may be different greens. For example, cilantro, tarragon or watercress. The main thing is that the leaves are young and non-rigid. And try to buy cheese that is as similar to parmesan as possible as or in any case not worse than it.

62. UNSWEETENED PIE WITH TOMATOES AND PARSLEY

INGREDIENTS

- mold butter
- yeast-free puff pastry - 250 g
- Medium bunch of parsley - 1 pc.
- 4-6 cherry tomatoes or 1 medium tomato
- Russian cheese - 50 g
- Olive oil - 1 tsp.
- salt, freshly ground black pepper

PREPARATION

1. Preheat oven to 180 ° C. Lubricate the round ceramic baking dish (diameter 15-18 cm) with butter.
2. Put dough on a flat surface and thaw. At this time, prepare the filling: wash the parsley and tomatoes, dry. Finely chop the leaves of parsley with a knife and put in a small bowl. Cherry cut into quarters, and if a large tomato, then diced. Grate the cheese.

3. Stretch out the dough a little with your hands so that it becomes rectangular. Put the cheese evenly on the dough, then parsley and tomatoes. Sprinkle the filling with olive oil, pepper and add a little bit of salt (the salt will be added by cheese). Roll up: it should turn out quite dense. Press the dough along the edges of the roll so that the filling does not fall out.
4. There are two options for baking a pie. In the first: you bake the whole roll, shifting it into a shape and folding it in the form of a "snail". In the second: roll should be cut into 7-8 pieces (about the same thickness of 3-4 cm). It is better to cut with a wide and sharp knife. Then shift the pieces of roll into the form, laying them out with the cut up. One piece to the center, and the rest to distribute around, like the petals of a flower - so it will be more convenient to eat it.
5. Bake the cake for 20 minutes. Serve warm by putting on a plate a piece of cake with a green salad dressed with olive oil.

63. VEGETABLE PIE WITH PARSLEY PESTO

INGREDIENTS

- 400 g puff pastry
- 150 g peas
- 1 red onion
- 2 carrots
- 1 zucchini
- 3 tbsp. l grated parmesan

For pesto:

- large bunch of parsley
- small bunch of basil
- 3/4 cup olive oil
- 3 tbsp. l pine nuts
- 3 cloves of garlic
- 1/2 tsp 5 pepper mixes
- salt to taste

PREPARATION

1. Rinse greens for pesto, dry, remove the stems. Grind the leaves with a knife. Crush in a mortar or whisk in a blender a uniform sauce of chopped leaves, nuts, chopped garlic, olive oil, pepper mixture and salt.
2. Cut zucchini and onions into half rings, carrots - in circles. Cut the pea pods in half. Mix vegetables with 2 tbsp. l pesto, cover with a film and leave for 1 hour.

3. Roll out the dough quite thinly (the thickness of the dough should not be more than 3-4 mm). Fold the edges of the dough in 2 turns, trimming the corners. Pound the dough with a fork. Put the remaining sauce first, then the vegetables.
4. Sprinkle with grated Parmesan and bake in the oven at 190 ° C for 20–25 minutes.

64. CABBAGE SOUP WITH CHICKEN

INGREDIENTS

- 1 head of young cabbage
- 2 large onions
- 1 head young garlic
- 1 small bunch of green onions
- 4–5 sprigs of parsley
- 2 chicken breast fillets
- 3 tbsp. l ghee
- Salt
- freshly ground black pepper

PREPARATION

1. Cut the chicken breast fillet as thinly as possible across the slices, salt and pepper.
2. Peel the onions and garlic. Cut the onion into very thin quarters of the rings, garlic into thin slices. Chop the cabbage finely by removing the stalk. Finely chop green onion and parsley.
3. In a large pan using a thick bottom, heat the melted butter; put the onions and garlic, fry over a low heat, stirring for 10 minutes. Add cabbage and green onions, fry for 2 minutes.

4. Pour in 1.2 liters of cold drinking water, bring to a boil over high heat, and cook under the lid, lowering the heat, 10 min. Salt. Add chicken and parsley, bring to a boil, turn off the heat, and insist under the lid for 10 minutes. Pepper and serve.

65. BLACK COD CONFIT WITH PARSLEY SALAD

INGREDIENTS

- 4 pieces of black cod fillet without skin, at least 2.5 cm thick, 120 g each
- 3-5 sprigs of parsley
- 2 rosemary shoots
- 1 liter of olive oil
- salt, black pepper to taste

For salad:

- 2 tbsp. l hazelnuts
- 10-12 sprigs of parsley
- 3-4 sprigs of green basil
- 2 tbsp. l olive oil
- 1 tsp lime juice
- 1 tsp. zest of lemon, lime and orange
- salt, black pepper to taste

PREPARATION

1. Put the black cod fillet in a pan of small diameter and about 7 cm deep. Add sprigs of parsley and rosemary and add cold olive oil. The oil should completely cover the fillet.
2. Heat the oil over very low heat to a temperature of 55 ° C (check the temperature with an electronic or alcohol kitchen thermometer) and cook at this temperature for about 20 minutes. Remove the oil fillet, pat dry with a napkin and season with salt and pepper.
3. For salad, chop parsley and basil leaves, mix with citrus zest, season with lemon juice and olive oil. If necessary, salt and pepper. Mix with coarsely chopped hazelnuts, mix.
Arrange the fillet on heated plates, serve the salad separately.

66. SLOW COOKED FISH SOUP WITH PARSLEY, POTATOES AND CORN

INGREDIENTS

- 500 g cod fillet
- 2 large

- bunches of parsley 1 onion
- 1 bunch of green onion
- 6 tbsp. l olive oil
- 2 cloves of garlic
- 4 potatoes
- 200 g of fresh or canned corn grains
- 100 ml cream with a fat content of 33%
- salt and pepper

PREPARATION

1. Prepare a slow cooker and ingredients.
2. Wash the parsley, dry and tear off the leaves from the stems. Peel and chop the garlic. Wash the potatoes, peel, cut into cubes. Rinse the fish and cut into portions. Chop onions finely.
3. Turn on the Multi-Cook mode, set the temperature to 160 ° C, warm the olive oil, fry the onions, 5 minutes, then add the garlic and potatoes. 5 minutes to cook
4. Pour 1.5 liters of water, bring to a boil and cook for 10 minutes. Chop the leaves of parsley and green onions and add to the soup along with fish and corn. Season with it salt and pepper, cook for 5 minutes.
5. Pour in the cream and mix.
6. Fish soup is ready.

67. CARROT SALAD WITH NUTS AND PARSLEY

INGREDIENTS

- 4–5 medium carrots
- 20 g of roasted hazelnuts and walnuts
- 1 medium bunch of parsley
- juice and zest of half a lemon
- unrefined olive oil or peanut butter
- 1 tbsp. l mustard seeds
- 0.5 tsp honey
- salt, freshly ground white pepper

PREPARATION

1. Peel off and grate the carrots on a coarse grater. In parsley, remove the stems. Chop the leaves very finely.
2. Mix lemon juice and zest with mustard, olive or peanut butter, salt, pepper and honey.
3. Chop the nuts - partly finely, partly larger. Mix carrots with parsley and nuts, pour dressing, mix and let stand for 15 minutes.

68. CHEESE AND PARSLEY PIE

INGREDIENTS

For filling:

- salt, black pepper
- Egg - 1 pc.
- bunch of parsley
- milk - 150 ml
- Russian cheese - 50 g
- Green onion feathers - 6 pcs.
- Yolk - 1 pc.

For the test:

- butter - 75 g
- flour - 175 g
- a pinch of salt

PREPARATION

1. Grind butter with sifted flour and salt. Add 2-3 tbsp. l cold water and knead the dough. Cover with plastic wrap up and then refrigerate for 30 minutes.
2. Grate the cheese. Wash onions and parsley and chop finely. In a bowl, mix the egg, yolk, cheese,

milk, onions and parsley, season with salt and pepper. To stir thoroughly.
3. Roll the dough in thin layer, put it into a mold. Spread the filling, cover with foil and bake in the oven at 200 ° C for 25 minutes. Remove foil and bake till golden brown, 5-7 minutes.

69. PARSLEY WITH GARLIC

INGREDIENTS

- parsley - 40 g
- crushed garlic - 4 cloves
- Flour - 450 g + 4 tbsp.
- pea flour - 50 g
- dry yeast - 7 g
- natural yogurt - 150 ml
- Salt - 0.5 tsp.
- Vegetable oil - 1 tbsp.
- Sesame seeds - 3 tbsp.

PREPARATION

1. Preheat the oven to 200 ° C, put a baking sheet inside so that it preheats. Wash the parsley, drain and chop finely, peel and chop the garlic. Sift flour, pea flour and yeast into a large bowl. Add parsley and garlic. Mix.
2. In a separate bowl, mix yogurt, vegetable oil and 150 ml of salted warm drinking water. The mixture should be at room temperature.
3. Pour the resulting mixture into dry ingredients and knead the dough. Knead on a powdery surface for

2 minutes. Return the dough inside a bowl, cover and leave for 10 minutes. At room temperature.
4. Hand knead the dough into a large cake, cut it into 4 sectors. Give each part a drop shape.
5. Stretch each cake 20 cm in length, trying to maintain the shape of the drop. Sprinkle cakes with water and sprinkle with sesame seeds. Put on a hot pan and bake for 7-8 minutes.

70. YOUNG POTATOES WITH GARLIC AND PARSLEY

INGREDIENTS

- Ground black pepper - to taste
- Parsley – optional
- Water (or broth) - 1 glass
- Salt to taste
- Small onions - 1 pc.
- Seasoning "Provencal herbs" - to taste
- Olive oil - 1-2 tbsp.
- Garlic - 1-2 cloves
- Large potatoes - 500 g

PREPARATION

1. Fry onion, garlic and herbs in a pan with a thick bottom, heat the oil, fry finely chopped onions until soft, add chopped parsley and chopped garlic, fry, stirring, for about 1 minute.
2. We clean young potatoes, Wash young potatoes thoroughly, you can lightly peel them.
3. Fry young potatoes with onions, garlic and herbs, Put the potatoes in a pan with onions, garlic and parsley, quickly fry, and pour water so that it covers the potatoes by 1/3. Salt, pepper, and add your favorite spices.
4. We cover up the pan with a lid and simmer young potatoes, Cover and simmer over low or medium heat for about 30 minutes; add water from time to time, if necessary. The potato is ready when it is completely soft.

71. SALSA VERDE WITH PARSLEY AND MINT

INGREDIENTS

- 40 g fresh parsley
- olive oil - 100 ml
- 20 g mint
- 1 slice of white bread
- Capers - 1 tbsp.
- garlic - 1 clove
- White wine vinegar - 1 tbsp.
- salt and pepper to taste

PREPARATION

1. Wash greens, dry. Peel and chop the garlic. Put greens, capers, garlic in a blender bowl, season with salt and pepper, add vinegar and chopped white bread. Grind to a homogeneous consistency.
2. Continuing to beat, pour inside a thin stream of olive oil.

72. TOMATOES STUFFED WITH SALMON AND CAPERS

INGREDIENTS

- Tomatoes - 2 pieces

- Salmon fillet - 450 g
- Capers - 1.5 tablespoons
- Olive oil - 3 tablespoons
- Parsley - 40 g
- Garlic - 2 cloves
- Breadcrumbs - 2 tablespoons
- Salt – taste
- Ground black pepper – taste

PREPARATION

1. Cut the tomatoes across in half and remove seeds and pulp with a sharp-edged spoon. Dry up tomatoes with a paper towel and set aside. (The pulp can be used for something else.)

2. Free the salmon from the skin and bones, cut into small cubes and put in a bowl. Cut capers, garlic, parsley and combine with salmon. Add one tablespoon of breadcrumbs, three tablespoons of olive oil, salt, pepper and mix.

3. Tightly stuff the tomatoes with a mixture of salmon, so that the top is a hill. Sprinkle with the remaining breadcrumbs and then drizzle with olive oil.

4. Put the tomatoes in a greased form and bake in an oven preheated to 200 degrees for about thirty-five minutes - or until they are browned.

73. SALAD WITH TUNA AND CAPERS

INGREDIENTS

- Green salad - ½ beam
- Canned tuna in its own juice - 120 g
- Cherry tomatoes - 10 pieces
- Pickled capers - 20 g
- Salt – taste
- Balsamic dressing – taste
- Cucumbers - 1 piece

PREPARATION

1. Tomatoes and cucumber cut into 4 parts, sectors. Break the salad, split the tuna into small pieces, and add capers, salt, mix.

2. Top with balsamic sauce.

74. SALMON TARTARE WITH CAPERS

INGREDIENTS

- Salmon fillets - 500 g
- Pickled capers - 1 tablespoon

- Shallot - 3 heads
- Chives - 1 bunch
- Freshly ground black pepper – taste
- Soy sauce - 1 tablespoon
- Lemon juice – taste
- Olive oil - 1 tablespoon

PREPARATION

1. Finely chop the salmon, approximately 0.5 centimeter cubes.

2. Very (!) Finely chop the shallots, chives (a little, it performs here rather a decorative function), capers.

3. Put everything in a bowl, add soy sauce, olive oil, and slightly sprinkle with lemon juice and pepper.

4. Gently mix. We put it in the molds and send it to the refrigerator for thirty minutes.

5. Then spread on plates with salad.

75. FLOUNDER WITH CAPER AND LEMON OIL

INGREDIENTS

- Flounder - 2 pieces
- Wheat flour - 85 g

- Olive oil - 3 tablespoons
- Sea salt – taste
- Ground black pepper – taste
- Butter - 50 g
- Capers - 50 g
- Lemon - ½ pieces
- Parsley - 40 g

PREPARATION

1. Roll the fish in flour mixed with salt and pepper.

2. Put a large frying pan with non-stick coating on a strong fire, pour out the oil and wait until it is heated. Put the fish in oil and shake the pan to make sure that the fish is not stuck. Leave the fish for 4 minutes until a golden crust appears, then turn the fish over and cook for another 4 minutes (without touching).

3. While the fish is cooking, prepare the oil from the capers and lemon. Heat a small skillet with medium heat, add oil and wait until it starts to bubble. After that, stir the oil with a wooden spoon until the foam begins to fall and turn brown. Quickly add capers, lemon juice and chopped parsley. Stir the mixture constantly. Remove from heat and do not refrigerate.

4. Once the fish is ready, put it on plates and pour hot oil on top with capers and lemon.

76. PASTA WITH TUNA AND CAPERS

INGREDIENTS

- Paste - 300 g
- Capers - 2 teaspoons
- Tuna - 100 g
- Olive oil – taste
- Bulb onions - 1 head
- Garlic - 2 cloves
- Salt – taste
- Ground black pepper – taste
- Tomatoes juice - 200 g

PREPARATION

1. Heat olive oil inside a frying pan, fry finely chopped onion and 2 cloves of garlic until transparent.

2. Add 200 grams of mashed tomatoes; boil for 5 minutes over low heat.

3. Add tuna and capers, simmer over low heat.

4. Cook the pasta.

5. Combine the paste and sauce, add salt and pepper to taste.

78. TOMATO SALAD WITH CAPERS

INGREDIENTS

- Roman tomatoes - 8 pieces
- Capers - 1.5 teaspoons
- Basil leaves - 4 pieces
- Olive oil - 3 teaspoons
- Garlic - 1 clove
- Honey - ¼ teaspoon
- Balsamic vinegar - 3 teaspoons

PREPARATION

1. Cut the tomatoes into quarters and extract the seeds. Preheat the grill and fry the tomatoes for 1-2 minutes on each side until characteristic stripes are formed and the tomatoes are soft. Leave to cool at room temperature and transfer to a bowl.

2. Combine capers, basil, butter, minced garlic and honey in a small bowl. Salt. Pour the tomatoes over the dressing

and mix well. The salad is served at room temperature with crispy bread and grilled meat.

79. NICOISE SALAD WITH FRESH TUNA, CAPERS AND ANCHOVIES

INGREDIENTS

- New potatoes - 8 pieces
- Olive oil - 130 ml
- Tuna fillet - 400 g
- Green beans - 180 g
- Garlic - 1 clove
- Dijon mustard - 1 teaspoon
- White wine vinegar - 2 tablespoons
- Lettuce leaves - 50 pieces
- Cherry tomatoes - 12 pieces
- Black olives - 90 g
- Capers - 2 tablespoons
- Anchovy fillet - 8 pieces
- Chicken egg - 2 pieces
- Lemon - 1 piece

PREPARATION

1. Boil the potatoes inside boiling salted water for about 10 minutes until tender. Drain, cut into small pieces and transfer to a bowl.
2. From the beans, cut the tails and cut into small pieces. Boil in boiling salted water for about 3 minutes, drain and rinse under cold water. Transfer to potatoes.
3. Heat olive oil inside a skillet over high heat. Cut the fish into small cubes and then fry in oil for about 3 minutes until golden brown. Transfer to vegetables.
4. Cook the eggs cool. Drain; dip in cold water for a while. Peel and cut into small pieces.
5. Mix chopped garlic, mustard and vinegar, then add the remaining olive oil, constantly stirring vigorously. Salt.
6. Put lettuce leaves on the bottom of the salad bowl. Lay on top the cooked salad, olives, half-sliced tomatoes and capers. Pour dressing and garnish with egg slices and anchovies. Pour lemon juice on top.

80. SALMON CARPACCIO WITH CAPERS

INGREDIENTS

- Tomatoes - 3 pieces
- Capers - 1 tablespoon
- Dill - 1 tablespoon
- Salmon fillets - 500 g
- Olive oil - 1 tablespoon
- Lime juice - 1 tablespoon
- Ciabatta - 1 piece

PREPARATION

1. Make a cross-shaped incision on top of the tomato. Transfer to a bowl and fill with boiling water. Leave on for 2-3 minutes. Transfer to ice water, dry and remove the skin. Cut into half, remove the seeds with a teaspoon and chop finely. Transfer to a bowl with capers and chopped dill. Mix well.

2. Using a sharp knife carefully cut the fish across the fibers into very thin pieces (the thinner the better). Arrange the fish in 4 plates in 1 layer.

3. Put a small amount of tomato mixture in the center of the plate. Whisk olive oil with lime juice, spices and salt. Sprinkle fish and tomatoes. Sprinkle generously with

freshly ground black pepper on top. Serve immediately with ciabatta.

81. PEPPERS STUFFED WITH TUNA AND CAPERS

INGREDIENTS

- Canned Tuna in Oil - 1 can
- Bell pepper - 4 pieces
- Chilli - ½ pieces
- Minced parsley - 2 tablespoons
- Pickled capers - 2 teaspoons
- Ground black pepper – taste
- Lemon juice - 3 tablespoons

PREPARATION

1. Gently peppers to remove from the stalk and seeds, rinse and place in the microwave for 3-4 minutes (or dip in boiling water for 8-9 minutes). Remove and lower in ice water. Carefully remove the skin without damaging the shape of the cones.

2. Prepare the filling: mix tuna, chili, capers and chopped parsley. Season with ground pepper and lemon juice.

3. Stuff the peppers with fish filling and cool.

82. VINAIGRETTE WITH CAPERS AND BAKED BEETS

INGREDIENTS

- Beet - 4 pieces
- Potatoes - 3 pieces
- Carrot - 2 pieces
- Salted cucumbers - 5 items
- Green pea - 1 can
- Sauerkraut - 150 g
- Pickled capers - 50 g
- Olive oil - 4 tablespoons
- Sea salt – taste
- Ground black pepper – taste
- Coarse sea salt - 50 g

PREPARATION

1. Wrap the beets in foil, pour a large sea in a baking sheet, not less than a centimeter, make a cut with a knife in each beet, wrapped, send to the oven for a couple of hours at 180-200 degrees.

2. Boil potatoes, it is important - do not digest. Boil carrots, it is important not to digest. Allow the vegetables to cool. Finely chop the cooked vegetables - the less chopped, the tastier, in my opinion (chopped into cubes).

3. Add canned green peas, I prefer small ones.

4. Finely chop sauerkraut. Peel pickles, chop into small cubes. Add capers.

5. Pour the resulting mass with olive oil, at least 3 tablespoons. Add salt and pepper to taste.

83. SALMON AND CAPER TARTARE

INGREDIENTS

- Salmon fillets - 250 g
- Capers - 1 teaspoon
- Chives - 1 bunch
- Lemon - ½ pieces
- Salt – taste
- Ground black pepper – taste
- Dill – taste

PREPARATION

1. First, cut the salmon fillet into thin slices, then into small cubes. Chopped capers washed and dried chives. Squeeze juice out of half a lemon.

2. In a bowl, gently mix the fish cubes with onions and lemon juice, add salt and black pepper to taste. Allow to stand for 8-10 minutes.

3. Carefully put the tartare on dessert plates or saucers, garnish with sprigs of dill.

84. SPAGHETTI WITH ANCHOVIES, PARSLEY, OLIVES AND CAPERS

INGREDIENTS

- Garlic - 2 cloves
- Minced parsley - 1.5 cups
- Bulb onions - 1 head
- Anchovies - 4 pieces
- Olives - ⅓ cup
- Capers - 2 teaspoons
- Ground black pepper - ¼ teaspoon
- Olive oil - ½ cup
- Spaghetti - 450 g
- Salt –taste

PREPARATION

1. Thoroughly grind garlic, parsley, onions, anchovies, pitted green olives in a food processor. Add salt (1/2 teaspoon), pepper, half a glass of olive oil and bring the mixture to a homogeneous state.

2. Boil water inside a large saucepan, add salt (2 teaspoons of salt to 8 liters of water) and throw pasta (spaghetti or linguine) there. Cook for 1 minute or indicated on the packet. Discard the finished pasta in a colander, drain the water and return the pasta to the pan.

3. Add 1 teaspoon of olive oil to pasta and mix. Transfer the pasta into a deep large dish, pour the cooked sauce with anchovies, mix thoroughly again and immediately serve.

85. BLUEBERRY PIE

INGREDIENTS

- Wheat flour - 1 cup
- Baking powder - 1 teaspoon
- Salt - 0.125 teaspoons
- Butter - 120 g
- Sugar - 1 cup
- Chicken egg - 2 pieces
- Blueberries - 400 g
- Lemon juice - ½ teaspoon
- Powdered sugar - 1 tablespoon

PREPARATION

1. Preheat the oven to 180 degrees. Oil a round shape (approximately 23 cm in diameter). Sprinkle with flour and shake off excess.

2. Sift the flour into a bowl, leaving 1 teaspoon, baking powder and salt.

3. In another bowl, beat the softened butter and sugar, leaving 1 teaspoon, until cream. Insert the eggs one at a time and beat again.

4. Whisk, add the oil mixture to the mixture with flour. Mix well and shift into shape.

5. In a bowl, combine blueberries, lemon juice, 1 teaspoon of flour and 1 teaspoon of sugar. Put the berries in an even layer on the dough and bake for about an hour until cooked.

6. Cool in a form and transfer to a dish, berries up. Sprinkle with powder and serve.

86. COTTAGE CHEESE CASSEROLE WITH BLUEBERRIES

INGREDIENTS

- Chicken egg - 2 pieces
- Brown sugar - 70 g
- Skim cheese - 600 g
- Semolina - 5 tablespoons
- Blueberries - 150 g

PREPARATION

1. Rub the yolks with a mixer with sugar and vanilla until white.

2. Add the cottage cheese and beat until smooth.

3. Pour semolina and mix blueberries.

4. Beat the whites and introduce into the mass.

5. Put in a greased mold and bake at 180 degrees 30 minutes.

87. BLUEBERRY MUFFINS

INGREDIENTS

- Blueberries - 200 g
- Wheat flour - 300 g
- Butter - 50 g
- Milk - 120 ml
- Chicken egg - 1 piece
- Sugar - 4 tablespoons
- Dry yeast - 15 g
- Salt – pinch

PREPARATION

1. Heat the milk a little (it should not boil), add sugar and dissolve the yeast in it. Leave it to stand 15 minutes inside a warm place without drafts.

2. Beat the egg and melted butter with a fork (most). Pour the egg mixture into the matching yeast. Mix gently. Knead the dough and leave to approach for an hour and a half.

3. Put the dough on the table, sprinkled with flour, roll into a layer with a thickness of about 10 mm. Grease with melted butter, and sprinkle with the remaining sugar. Spread the blueberries over the entire surface of the dough, and then press the berries in with a rolling pin. Roll them into a roll, and then cut into pieces about 2 cm thick. Turnover, flatten a little by hand and fold on a greased baking sheet so that they touch each other. Cover with a towel and let it go for about 20 minutes.

4. Bake in a preheated oven to 180 degrees until cooked. Serve warm.

88. BLUEBERRY YOGURT BANANA SMOOTHIE

Energy Value Per Portion

- Calorie Content: 299 Kcal
- Squirrels: 9,4 Gram
- Fats: 3.8 Gram
- Carbohydrates: 58.4 Gram

Ingredients

- Bananas - 1 piece
- Orange juice - ½ cup
- Natural yogurt - ½ cup
- Blueberries - ¼ cup

PREPARATION

1. Cut the banana in small pieces and freeze.

2. in a blender, mix banana, yogurt, orange juice and blueberries. Grind until smooth and pour into a tall glass.

89. BLUEBERRY AND CINNAMON MUFFINS

INGREDIENTS

- Wheat flour - 435 g
- Baking powder - 2 teaspoons
- Salt - 1 teaspoon
- Cinnamon - ¾ teaspoon
- Sugar - 180 g
- Butter - 80 g
- Fat milk - 230 ml
- Chicken egg - 3 pieces
- Blueberries - 100 g

PREPARATION

1. Heat the oven to 180 degrees. Put 18 paper muffin baking tins on two or three muffin baking tins.

2. Sift flour inside a large bowl; add baking powder, salt and cinnamon. Stir and pour sugar. Rub in unsalted butter with a fork until the mixture resembles crumbs.

3. Using a fork, beat milk and egg together in a mug. Gently pour this liquid into the flour mixture, then beat and add blueberries with a spatula with a rubber tip.

4. Fill the paper molds with two-thirds pastry. Bake muffins in the center of the oven for 25 minutes, until they rise and turn golden brown. Leave them in paper for a few minutes, and then remove the paper and transfer to the grate. Serve either warm or immediately after cooking.

90. BLUEBERRY DUMPLINGS

Energy Value Per Portion

- Calorie Content: 780 Kcal
- Squirrels: 25.8 Gram
- Fats: 8.3 Gram
- Carbohydrates: 152.5 Gram

Ingredients

- Kefir - 1 cup
- Wheat flour - 4 cups
- Chicken egg - 3 pieces
- Blueberries – taste
- Sugar – taste
- Salt – pinch
- Butter – taste
- Soda – pinch

Preparation

1. Stir kefir and eggs well, add soda, salt and flour (3-4 cups), knead steep dough. Cover up the dough with a bowl and let stand for about 30 minutes.
2. Cut a piece from the dough, shape it into a sausage with a diameter of about 2 cm, cut the sausage

into pieces about 1-1.5 cm thick. Dip each piece into flour on both sides and roll it into a circle.
3. In the middle of each cup put half a teaspoon of blueberries mixed with sugar, carefully pinch the edges.
4. Boil dumplings in slightly salted water for about 10 minutes after boiling. Before serving, you can sprinkle with sugar, sour cream or cream, or pour over melted butter.

91. OATMEAL WITH BANANA AND BLUEBERRIES

Energy Value Per Portion

- Calorie Content: 204 Kcal
- Squirrels: 6.5 Gram
- Fats: 3.3 Gram
- Carbohydrates: 38.1 Gram

Ingredients

- Blueberries - 250 g
- Kefir - 150 ml
- Cereals - 80 g
- Ground cinnamon – taste
- Bananas - 150 g
- Vanillin – taste

PREPARATION

1. Pour oatmeal with kefir.

2. Add banana and blueberries (you can beat everything in a blender).

3. Add vanillin and cinnamon to the cream to taste.

4. Put in glasses, garnish with banana slices and blueberries on top.

92. BLUEBERRIES WITH COTTAGE CHEESE AND HONEY

INGREDIENTS

- Cottage cheese - 400 g
- Frozen blueberries - 1 kg
- Buckwheat honey - 3 tablespoons
- Green pistachios - 100 g
- Sugar - 100 g
- Cream 35% - 500 ml
- Gelatin in plates - 4 pieces

PREPARATION

1. Turn blueberries into mashed potatoes in a blender. Beat cream with sugar and mix with blueberry puree. Soak gelatin in water, squeeze water and mix gelatin with cream and blueberries.

2. Cottage cheese mixed with honey. At the bottom of each of the six molds put a layer of cottage cheese and pour a mixture of cream and blueberries. Refrigerate and hold until mixture thickens. When serving, sprinkle with chopped pistachios.

93. CHOCOLATE CAKE WITH BLUEBERRIES AND CHERRIES

INGREDIENTS

- Cherry - 400 g
- Blueberries - 150 g
- Cherry liquor - 4 tablespoons
- bitter chocolate - 400 g
- Butter - 150 g
- Chicken egg - 4 pieces
- Sugar - 175 g
- Wheat flour - 75 g
- Cream - 500 ml

PREPARATION

1. Put the cherries and blueberries in a bowl with 3 tablespoons of liquor, cover and let it brew for about 3 hours.
2. Preheat the oven to 180 degrees. Melt 100 grams of chocolate in a water bath. Remove, let cool slightly and add the yolks, the remaining liquor and beat thoroughly.
3. Beat butter with sugar. Combine with the chocolate mixture, and then add the flour.
4. Separately, beat the whites and add to the chocolate dough and mix.
5. Put the dough in a baking dish, padded with parchment and greased with oil. Bake for 25-30 minutes.

6. Melt chocolate and combine with cream. Bring the chocolate mixture to a boil, stirring constantly. Allow to cool.
7. Put the berries on a biscuit, pour over the juice. Spread chocolate cream mixture on top with a spoon and smooth. Garnish with fresh berries.
8. Put the finished cake in the refrigerator for 2 hours.

94. BLUEBERRY AND BANANA SMOOTHIE

Energy Value Per Portion

- Calorie Content: 202 Kcal
- Squirrels: 4.9 Gram
- Fats: 1.8 Gram
- Carbohydrates: 43.5 Gram

Ingredients

- Lime - ½ g
- Frozen blueberries - 300 g
- Oranges - 4 pieces
- Rice Vanilla Milk - 1 cup
- Bananas - 1 piece
- Cereals - 3 tablespoons

PREPARATION

1. Defrost blueberries on the top shelf of the refrigerator or you can put frozen - then the smoothie will be cold.

2. Squeeze the juice from half lime and 4 oranges; if you like acidic, you can take a whole lime.

3. Peel and chop the banana coarsely.

4. Put blueberries, banana, juice in a blender and add oatmeal and a glass of rice milk (you can replace it with ordinary).

5. Punch everything at high speed.

6. Serve. Garnishing with mint leaves.

95. TURMERIC LENTIL SOUP

INGREDIENTS

- Garlic - 3 cloves
- Red lentils - 300 g
- Ginger - 50 g
- Turmeric - 2 teaspoons
- Asafoetida - 1 teaspoon
- Salt – taste
- Cream - 100 ml
- Tomatoes - 1 piece
- Carrot - 2 pieces
- Bulb onions - 1 piece

PREPARATION

1. Soak lentils overnight. For soups and stews it is better to take red Persian lentils or yellow - they are better than others boiled. Soak lentils for this reason: all legumes contain phytic acid, which makes it difficult for heaps of useful substances like calcium to enter our body and complicates metabolism. Soaking removes this problem.
2. Boil the lentils for an hour.
3. While it is cooking: chop the onion, chop the tomato, peeling it off (just hold it under boiling

water for 10 minutes), grate the carrots on a coarse grater and ginger on a fine grater.
4. Fry the vegetables by adding them to the pan with a difference of 5 minutes in this order: onions, carrots, ginger, and tomato.
5. Next, add seasonings. There are two ways to do this. The first one is longer: put butter, squeezed garlic, and turmeric and asafetida on the bottom of a clean pan. Seasonings fried in butter reveal their aromas better. So that they do not burn, pour cream into the butter. And then lentils, from which we pre-drain the water. The second way: if you are too lazy to stain another pan, you can drain the water from the lentils, add cream and add all these seasonings immediately to the lentils.
6. Cook lentils with seasonings for another 20 minutes.
7. Put vegetables in lentils. Boil another 10 minutes.
8. Grind everything turned out in a blender.
9. Serve with pumpkin seeds and toasted bread.

96. TURMERIC AND BASIL CARROT PUREE

INGREDIENTS

- Carrot - 500 g
- Grape Seed Oil - 50 ml
- Green basil - ½ beam
- Ground Cumin (Zira) - ½ teaspoon
- Turmeric - 1 teaspoon
- Salt – taste
- Ground black pepper – taste

PREPARATION

1. 500 grams of carrots, peel and cut across into 1 cm thick bars
2. Fill with water and cook until cooked. We check readiness like a potato with a knife
3. Put the carrots in the harvester, add grape seed oil (it is neutral and will not clog other tastes such as olive) leaves and stalks of basil postponing a few ground cumin and turmeric for decoration
4. Salt and pepper to taste
5. Punch everything until smooth, if necessary adding grape seed oil
6. Sprinkle with fresh basil leaves on top
7. Serve as a side dish

97. STRAWBERRY MOUSSE CURD CAKE

INGREDIENTS

Dough:

- Butter - 150 g
- Egg - 2 pcs.
- Sugar - 100 g
- Baking powder - 1 tsp
- Wheat flour - 350 g
- Salt - a pinch

Curd filling:

- Soft curd - 500 g
- Sugar - 100 g
- Vanilla Sugar - 10 g
- Sour cream - 3 tablespoons
- Eggs - 2 pcs.
- Starch - 2-3 tbsp.

Strawberry Mousse:

- Strawberry - 400 g
- Sugar - 120 g
- Starch - 2 tbsp.

PREPARATION
1. Put soft butter inside a bowl and add sugar and salt, whisk with a whisk.
2. Then add eggs and continue whipping.
3. Sift in parts flour together with baking powder.
4. Knead soft dough. While the filling is to be prepared, the dough must be put in a plastic bag and put in the refrigerator.
5. Put soft cottage cheese, ordinary and vanilla sugar, starch and sour cream in a blender bowl.
6. Beat the whole mass until smooth.
7. Add eggs to the bowl and beat again.
8. For strawberry mousse, wash strawberries, tear tails and put in a saucepan, add sugar.
9. Puree strawberries with a hand blender. Add starch to the strawberry puree and mix thoroughly so that there are no lumps.
10. Put the mass on the fire and cook until thickened. The mass should remain pouring.
11. From the refrigerator, get the dough, roll it to fit the shape (I have 24 cm), and make 4 cm high sides. Pour the curd filling onto the dough. Then gently pour strawberry mousse on top.
12. Preheat oven to 180 degrees and bake the cake for 50-55 minutes. The cake must be completely

cooled in shape, and then put in the refrigerator for several hours or overnight.
13. Curd pie with strawberry mousse is incredibly delicious! Cut it into portions with sharp knife and serve.

98. JELLY CANDIES

INGREDIENTS

- Frozen Berries - 400-450 g
- Instant gelatin - 40 g
- Sugar - 300 g
- Lemon (juice) - 1 pc.
- Coconut flakes - 3-4 pinches
- Vegetable oil - to lubricate the mold

PREPARATION

1. Prepare a container for cooling the jelly mass - line with baking paper, grease with oil and sprinkle with coconut.
2. Sprinkle the frozen berries with sugar and thaw. Make a mixture of strawberries (200 g), raspberries

(200 g) and black currant (1 handful), but one kind of berries is enough.
3. To speed up the process, you can unfreeze the berries in a microwave or install a bowl of berries in a water bath.
Grind the resulting mixture of berries, juice and sugar to a puree state.
4. Pour the resulting fruit puree into the pan. Add lemon juice and instant gelatin.
5. On a small fire, warm the mixture for several minutes, stirring constantly, until the gelatin and sugar dissolve. If necessary, you can bring the mixture to a boil and turn off the fire immediately.
6. When the gelatin dissolves, turn off the heat and cool the mixture to a temperature of 36-37 degrees. To ensure the mixture has cooled sufficiently, drop a drop of fruit mass on your hand. If it is not felt on the skin, the temperature is correct.
7. Beat the mixture with a mixer for 8-10 minutes until it brightens and doubles in volume.
8. Pour the mixture inside the prepared container and place in the refrigerator for 3-4 hours for final cooling.
9. When the mixture cools and solidifies completely, remove it from the mold.

10. Pour boiling water over the knife blade, pat it dry with a napkin, and cut the jelly mass into pieces of the desired size. If desired, roll the resulting sweets with powdered sugar. Store sweets in the refrigerator in an airtight container.

99. PIE "STRAWBERRY DELIGHT"

INGREDIENTS

- Butter - 50 g
- Vegetable oil - 50 g
- Milk - 150 ml.
- Sugar - 170 g
- Vanilla Sugar - 1 sachet
- Flour - 250 g
- Dough baking powder - half a bag
- Egg - 2 pcs.
- Strawberries - 500 g
- Coconut flakes - 4 tbsp.
- Powdered sugar - 3 tbsp.

PREPARATION

1. Beat eggs with sugar until white.
2. 300 grams of strawberries cut into halves and fall asleep 2 tbsp. Coconut
3. In beaten eggs, add melted butter and vegetable oil, as well as milk. Stir. Next, add the flour and baking powder. Mix everything well again and pour into a mold with a diameter of 26 centimeters, greased with oil.

4. Now spread our strawberries on top. And sprinkle with coconut on top
5. Put in the oven for 45 minutes, bake at 180 degrees.
6. Ready, cooled cake on top decorates with the remaining strawberries, cut in half. Pour it with icing sugar mixed with a spoonful of water. You can just sprinkle with powdered sugar; it is at your discretion.

100. STRAWBERRY CAKE "CLOUD"

INGREDIENTS

- Cookies - 150 g
- Coconut Chips - 0.5 cups
- Butter - 100 g
- Ground cinnamon - 0.5-1 tsp
- Egg white - 2 pcs.
- Sugar - 1 cup or slightly less (to taste)
- Strawberry - 250 g
- Lemon juice - 1 tbsp.
- Vanilla or vanilla sugar to taste

Additionally:

- Cardamom - 4-6 boxes

PREPARATION

1. Grind cookies with a blender or rolling pin.
2. Combine chopped cookies and coconut. Add cinnamon, melted butter and mix well.
3. Cover the bottom of the detachable shape with parchment paper.
4. Put the cookie mixture into the mold. Flatten by pressing with a spoon or fingers. The base should not be thick; otherwise, when it hardens in the freezer, to cut it, you will have to try. It is enough that it only covers the bottom of the form with a continuous even thin layer.
5. Place the cake pan in the refrigerator or freezer to cool.
6. Now let's prepare the very "cloud". Take a large bowl - the mixture will greatly increase in volume. Combine egg whites, sugar, strawberries, lemon juice and vanilla. If possible, add some ground cardamom - an incredibly tasty combination.
7. Beat everything first until smooth, and then continue to whisk until the mixture has tripled in volume. Use room temperature proteins to speed up the process.

Rub a drop of protein mass with your fingertips, sugar grains should not be felt.
8. Put the protein mixture on the cooled cake and smooth.
9. Place in the freezer for 4 hours. While the cake is cooling, in addition to it, you can make quick strawberry sauce.
10. Strawberry Cake "Cloud" is ready! Decorate the finished cake as desired. Store the cake in the freezer. In a sealed container, the cake can be stored for up to 1 month.
11. Cut the cake, after dipping the blade of the knife in hot water for a few seconds. In the freezer, the cake cools and hardens. But it will become airy and tender, like a cloud, after only a few minutes at room temperature.

101. Strawberry Curd Cupcakes

INGREDIENTS

- Cottage cheese - 250 g
- Butter - 120 g

- Chicken eggs - 2 pcs.
- Sugar - 200 g
- Soda - 0.5 tsp
- Wheat flour - 250 g
- Strawberry - 150 g

PREPARATION

1. Hammer eggs in a bowl and add sugar.
2. Beat eggs using sugar using a mixer until smooth and fluffy.
3. Melt the butter inside water bath or microwave, cool and add to the egg mixture. Once again, beat everything with a mixer.
4. Add cottage cheese and mix (cottage cheese of any fat content is suitable for this recipe).
5. Pour the sifted flour with soda and mix again.
6. The dough will turn out quite thick, but at the same time soft and not clogged.
7. Put the dough in muffin tins. If you bake cupcakes in metal molds, grease them with butter, silicone does not need to be lubricated. During baking, the dough rises well, so do not fill the molds to the top.
8. Wash strawberries well, dry and remove the stalks. Put a berry in each tin, squeezing it a little in the dough.

9. Send the cupcakes to the oven preheated to 180 degrees and bake until they are a beautiful golden color (25-30 minutes). The baking time depends on your oven.
10. Remove the prepared curd muffins with strawberries from the mold and let them cool completely.

102. Strawberry Sponge Cake

INGREDIENTS

- Vegetable oil - 50 ml.
- Vanillin - 1 g
- Sugar - 5 tbsp.
- Eggs - 3 pcs.
- Food coloring - 0.125 g
- Wheat flour - 1 cup
- Baking powder - 1 tsp.
- Strawberry puree - 80 g
- Salt - 1 pinch

Cream:

- Powdered whipped cream - 1 packet (30 g)
- Milk - 65 ml.

- Cream (20%) - 65 ml.

Strawberry Smoothie:
- Frozen Strawberries - 150 g
- Powdered sugar - 2 tbsp. l

Decoration and impregnation:
- Strawberry puree - 80 g
- Black Chocolate - 100 g
- Butter - 20 g

PREPARATION

1. Separately, in a bowl, mix all the dry ingredients - flour, half sugar, necessarily salt, several crystals of dry dye, baking powder and vanillin.
2. Large eggs are divided into proteins and yolks. Beat the whites with half the remaining sugar and a pinch of salt. Grind the yolks with a whisk. Punch strawberries in a blender with powdered sugar. You cannot defrost it. Mashed potatoes are divided into two parts.
3. Add half the strawberry puree to the yolks, pour in the vegetable oil and stir well. We use only a hand whisk. Then gradually pour the whole dry mixture with flour. Do not immediately stir all the flour, leave a couple of spoons; otherwise it will turn out

too thick. In several stages, mix whipped proteins to the strawberry mass. This is best done with a spatula.
4. It is necessary to try to interfere with proteins only in one direction, so as not to lose air bubbles. Do not rub anything. Put magnificent dough on a baking sheet with parchment. Bake for 12 -13 minutes at 180 degrees.
5. Carefully peel off the finished biscuit from the paper, prying it with a spatula and roll it up with a tight roll using the same parchment.
6. Allow the roll to cool completely when folded.
7. Meanwhile, prepare any cream. I whipped powdered cream-cream from a pack with milk. Unroll the roll and grease the surface with strawberry puree.
8. Then spread with whipped cream. And again tightly wrap in a roll. Let it cool for several hours.
9. To decorate, grease the surface of the roll with melted chocolate with butter or decorate as desired.

103. SALAD WITH STRAWBERRIES, MOZZARELLA AND ARUGULA

INGREDIENTS

- Fresh strawberries - 300 g
- Arugula - 100 g
- Mozzarella Cheese - 250 g
- Salt to taste
- Balsamic cream to taste
- Olive oil to taste
- Ground black pepper - to taste

PREPARATION

1. Wash strawberries, dry with a paper towel and cut in half.
2. Dice the cheese.
3. Place the arugula at the bottom of the salad bowl.
4. Top with mozzarella and strawberries.
5. Salad and pepper to taste. Sprinkle with olive oil and balsamic cream.
6. Salad with strawberries, mozzarella and arugula is ready. Serve chilled.

104. STRAWBERRY JAM TART

INGREDIENTS

Dough:

- Flour - 350-400 g

- Butter (frozen) - 200 g
- Sugar - 40 g
- Baking powder - 10 g
- Egg (large) - 1 pc.
- Salt - a pinch
- Vanillin - to taste

Filling:

- Strawberry Jam - 400 g

PREPARATION

1. Pour baking powder into flour, stir.
2. Grate the butter, add to the flour and grind to the state of crumbs.
3. Add sugar, salt, vanillin to the egg and beat with a mixer.
4. Pour the whipped mass into a mixture of flour and oil.
5. Knead the dough. The dough will turn out plastic and not sticky.
6. Weigh the dough and divide it into 3 equal parts. Two-thirds of the test will go to the base, 1/3 of the test - to the decoration. For a pie, you need a mold with a diameter of 20-22 cm. Cover the bottom of the mold using baking paper. Spread 2/3

of the dough on the bottom of the mold, making low sides.
7. Spread thick strawberry jam evenly on the base of the dough.
8. Bend the sides of the dough to the filling. Roll out a layer 0.3-0.5 cm thick from the rest of the dough, cut out the decoration using cookie cutters and place them on the surface of the cake. Bake the cake inside an oven preheated to 180 degrees for about 20-30 minutes, until lightly browned. Chill and cut into slices.

105. STRAWBERRY BANANA SMOOTHIE

INGREDIENTS

- Strawberries - 400-500 g
- Banana - 2 pcs.
- Milk - 500 ml
- Sugar / honey – optional

PREPARATION

1. Wash the strawberries and remove the stalks.
2. Peel off and cut the bananas into small slices.
3. Put the fruit in the blender bowl. If desired, add 1-2 tbsp. sugar (adjust the level of sugar, depending

on the sweetness of the fruit and your own taste preferences).
4. Beat the ingredients for several minutes until a smoothie is smooth. Add milk and whisk still 1-2 minutes at high speed
5. Pour the drink into glasses, decorate according to your mood and serve to the table.

106. Creamy Strawberry cup

For one person

Preparation time: 10 mins

Freezing time: 30 mins

To make this delicious ice cream we need:

Ingredients:

- 500 gr of very ripe raspberries
- 25 cl of cooking cream
- 235 gr of sugar

Preparation:

All you have to do put all the ingredients in the blender, and we are going to beat it little by little until you achieve the desired texture, and then put it in the freezer in a silicone mold, leave it in at least 30 minutes.

Nutritional Information

- 20% Total Fat 13g
- 41% Saturated Fat 8.2g.
- Trans Fat 0g
- 18% Cholesterol 53mg
- 4% Sodium 96mg
- 7% Potassium 262mg
- 10% Total Carbohydrates 30g
- 7% Dietary Fiber 1.8g

107. Apple Green Ceviche

3 Servings

Preparation time: 10 minutes

Cooking time: 20 minutes

Ingredients

- 1/4 cup of lemon juice
- 1/3 cup of orange juice
- 2 tablespoons of olive oil
- 1/4 bunch of cilantro
- 2 pieces of green apple without peel, cut into medium cubes
- 1 piece of finely chopped serrano chili
- 1 cup of jicama cut into medium cubes
- 1 piece of avocado cut into cubes
- 1 cup cucumber cut into cubes
- 1/4 bunch of finely chopped basil leaf
- 1/4 cup of finely chopped cilantro
- 1 pinch of salt
- 1 piece of sliced radish
- 1 piece of serrano chili cut into slices
- 1/4 piece of purple onion

Preparation

1. Add lemon juice, orange juice, olive oil and cilantro to the blender. Blend perfectly well. Reservation.
2. Add to a bowl the apple, serrano pepper, jicama, avocado, cucumber, basil, cilantro, mix with the preparation of the blender and season perfectly well.
3. Serve the ceviche in a deep dish and decorate with the radish the chile serrano and the purple onion. Enjoy

Nutritional information

- Percentage of daily values based on a 2,000-calorie diet.
- Calories   61.9   kcal 3.1%
- Carbohydrates   14.4   g 4.8%
- Proteins   1.6   g 3.1%
- Lipids   0.3   g 0.4%
- Dietary fiber   5.1   g 10%
- Sugars   6.2   g 6.9%
- Cholesterol   0.0   mg 0.0%

108. Soup 'green

Quantity: 1 person

Preparation: 15 minutes

Refrigeration: 15 minutes (optional)

Ingredients:

Water in sufficient quantity to achieve the desired texture

1 green apple with skin

1 slice of fresh peeled ginger

Half lemon or 1 lime without skin, the white part without seeds

Half cucumber with skin

Half bowl of leaves with fresh spinach

1 bunch of basil or fresh cilantro

1 branch of wireless celery, including tender green leaves

Preparation:

1. Wash and chop all the ingredients. Insert them into the glass of blender and crush.

2. Add the water and crush again until you get a homogeneous texture. If necessary, rectify water.

3. Take the soup as a snack at any time of the day to purify the body and keep cravings at bay. To know more: This cold soup is quick to prepare and has great benefits for the body. Perhaps the best-known property of the apple is its intestinal regulatory action. If we eat it raw and with skin, it is useful to treat constipation, since this way we take advantage of its richness in insoluble fiber present in the skin, which stimulates the intestinal activity and helps to keep the intestinal muscles in shape. Also, green apples are one of the largest sources of flavonoids. These antioxidant compounds can stop the action of free radicals on the cells of the body. Eating raw fruits and vegetables is the healthiest option.

Nutritional Information

    Calories 330

    Fat 12 g 18 %

    Cholesterol 90 mg

    Sodium 240 mg 10 %

    Carbohydrate 20 g 6 %

    Fibre 5 g 22 %

    Sugars 4 g

Iron 15 %

109. Stuffed Zucchini

Preparation: 15 min

45 min cooking

Total: 1 h: 3

Serves: 1-2 People

Ingredients

2 small red onions

2 small brown peppers

2 small round zucchini

3 cloves garlic, minced

300 grams of chopped mushrooms

1 chopped carrot

2 teaspoons paprika

2 teaspoons dried marjoram

1 teaspoon dried thyme

300 grams of cooked lentils

120 ml of fried tomato

1 teaspoon salt and more to splash the vegetables

Pepper

Preparation

Preheat the oven to 200 ° C.

Cut the tops of the vegetables and take out the interiors with a spoon. Chop the interiors of zucchini and onions.

Heat a pan over medium high heat and add the inside of the onions, garlic and a water jet (you can use oil). Once poached, add the mushrooms and fry until golden brown. Add the carrot and the inside of the zucchini. Fry until soft and the liquid has evaporated.

Add the paprika and herbs and fry a few seconds to release the aroma. Add the lentils, fried tomatoes, salt and pepper and cook a few minutes so that the flavors are mixed.

Season the interiors of the empty vegetables and fill with the lentils. Place them on a tray and return their covers. Bake 45 to 60 minutes or until easily punctured with a knife.

Take view from time to time and if the covers start to burn, or remove or cover with silver paper;

Let cool a few minutes before serving.

Nutritional Value

Amount per Serving

Calories: 245 kcal

 % Daily Values*

Total Fat4.24g7%

Saturated Fat1.915g10%

Trans Fat-

Polyunsaturated Fat0.245g

Monounsaturated Fat1.654g

Cholesterol12mg4%

Sodium169mg7%

Total Carbohydrate3.14g1%

Dietary Fiber0.2g1%

Sugars0.4g

Protein4.56g

110. Pumpkins with Quinoa

Preparation: 5 mins

Cooking Time: Approx. 20 mins

Number of Serving: 2

Ingredients

- ✓ 2 medium violin pumpkins
- ✓ 150 g of tricolor quinoa
- ✓ 200 g cooked chickpeas
- ✓ 30 g of pine nuts
- ✓ 40 g of blueberries
- ✓ Dried reds
- ✓ A few sprigs of parsley
- ✓ 4 tablespoons extra virgin olive oil
- ✓ Salt
- ✓ Pepper
- ✓ 1 teaspoon turmeric
- ✓ 100 g fresh spinach

Preparation

Cut the pumpkins in half lengthwise and, with the help of a spoon, remove the seeds. Place them inside baking dish lined with sulfurized paper and cook in the preheated oven at 200 degrees for 1 hour. Click with a knife to check that they are well cooked, remove from the oven and let it temper.

Wash the quinoa. In a saucepan, boil plenty of salt water and add the quinoa. Cook 20 minutes, drain and reserve. With the assistance of a spoon, empty the pumpkins, leaving a little pulp so as not to break the peel.

Heat a pan with olive oil, add the chopped pumpkin pulp, quinoa, cooked and drained chickpeas, pine nuts, cranberries, and chopped parsley. Season with salt, pepper and small turmeric. Sauté a couple of minutes and, finally, add fresh spinach. Saute one more minute and remove from heat. Fill the pumpkins with the mixture, sprinkle with a pinch of turmeric and serve.

Nutritional Value:

Calories: 190.

Sugar: 6.4g.

Fat: 6g.

Carbohydrates: 27.3g.

Fiber: 6.8g.

Protein: 7g.

111. Pea salad, gourmet peas, grapefruit

A fresh, crunchy and fruity starter.

6 People

Preparation Time: 20 Min

Cooking Time: 10 Min

Calories: 1 Cal / Pers.

Ingredients

1 pink grapefruit

800 g shelled peas

200 g gourmet peas

2 fresh onions with the stem

1 tray of sprouted seeds

1 drizzles of olive oil

1 dash of apple cider vinegar

1 tablespoon old-fashioned mustard

Seeds sesame toasted

PREPARATION

1. Peel the grapefruit and collect the flesh (without the white skin), as well as the juice.

2. Steam peas 3-4 minutes and gourmet peas a little more.

3. Mix the mustard in a salad bowl with the grapefruit juice, olive oil, vinegar, salt and pepper. Add the chopped onions with the stem, the vegetables and the grapefruit flesh. Mix well, sprinkle with sesame and sprinkle with sprouted seeds.

112. Indian pea dip

A vegan dip that has it all.

4 People

Preparation Time: 10 Min.

Ingredients

200 g frozen peas

2 tablespoon (s) of coriander

2 tablespoon (s) of mint

1 chopped green pepper

2 organic limes

2 tablespoon (s) of coconut cream

Salt pepper

Preparation

1. Cover 200 g of frozen peas with boiling water.

2 In a bowl, mix 2 tsp. coriander and 2 tsp. minced mint, chopped green pepper, zest of 2 organic limes, juice of 1 lime, 2 tsp. coconut cream, salt and pepper.

3 Mash the drained peas; mix them with the rest of the ingredients.

113. Millet veggie kale Paupiettes, apple pear chutney

A veggie dish that heats up in the dead of winter.

4 People

Preparation Time: 40 Mins.

Cooking Time: 75 Min.

Ingredients

1 large cabbage kale

300 g millet or quinoa

2 onions.2 cloves of garlic

2 multicolored carrots

1 celery stalk

2 sprigs of parsley

1/2 teaspoon curry powder

4 tablespoon (s) of olive oil

1 l hot vegetable or poultry broth

For the chutney

2 pears

2 apples.1 onion.

the juice of 1 orange

25 g peeled and grated ginger

3 tablespoon (s) of apple cider vinegar

2 tablespoons (s) soup sugar cane

Preparation

1. Blanch the 12 largest cabbage leaves for 10 minutes in a casserole dish of salted boiling water. Drain them; pass them under cold water, then remove the central rib if it is thick.

2. Rinse the millet or quinoa, and then cook it for 8 minutes in boiling salted water. Drain it. Chop the parsley. Peel and chop the onions. Peel, peel and chop the garlic cloves. Peel the carrots and cut them into brunoise. Chop the celery. Heat the olive oil inside a Dutch oven, and brown the onions, garlic, carrots, celery and curry for 15 minutes over low heat. Add salt and pepper. Mix the quinoa or millet and the vegetables.

3. Preheat the oven to 180 ° / th. 6. Stuff the cabbage leaves with the cereal-vegetable mixture and form small packages. Tie them. Store the paupiettes in a baking dish, drizzle with broth and cook for 20 to 30 minutes with small simmers. Lower the temperature if the lids start to color.

4. For the chutney, peel and seed the pears and apples. Cut them into pieces. Peel and chop the onion. Gather all the ingredients inside a saucepan and cook for about 20 minutes. Let cool.

5. Serve the paupiettes with a little cooking broth and the chutney aside.

114. Broad beans, peas, gourmet peas and mint

A chef's dish to endlessly use spring products.

4 People

Preparation Time: 30 Min.

Cooking Time: 30 Min

Ingredients

1.8 kg peas (800 g shelled)

1.2 kg of beans (375 g shelled)

400 g gourmet peas.10 g sugar

25 cl + 1/2 teaspoon (s) Coffee white balsamic vinegar

50 g pea sprouts

50 g sagebrush

1 onion withers

1 cl olive oil

1 bunch of mint

60 cl milk

Preparation

1. Shell the peas and beans. Bring 1.5 l of salted water to a boil in a saucepan, add the pea pods and cook for 10 minutes. Remove them with a skimmer. Add the peas to the broth, and then cook for 3 to 4 minutes. Take out the peas with a skimmer and cool them in ice water.

2. Mix 2/3 of the peas with 50 cl of cooking broth to obtain a soup. Reserve 1/3 of the peas and the remaining cooking broth.

3. Place the chopped mint in a saucepan, add the milk, and bring to the boil. Remove from the heat, let steep for 30 minutes, filter and set aside. Dip the gourmet peas 2 to 3 minutes in a saucepan of boiling salted water, then the beans 1 to 2 minutes. Let them cool in ice water. Remove the skin from the beans.

4. Reduce 25 cl of balsamic vinegar until you get a syrupy juice. In the reserved cooking broth, heat the beans, the 1/3 peas and the gourmet peas for 2 to 3 minutes.

5. Heat and froth the mint milk. Heat the pea soup; add a few sprouts of peas and sagebrush, season with olive oil and the rest of the white balsamic vinegar.

6. In a deep plate, pour the pea soup, add the beans, gourmet peas and drained peas. Add the chopped sweet onion, the sugar, the rest of the pea and sagebrush sprouts, the reduced vinegar and the frothed mint milk.

115. Broccoli, Zucchini & Onions Soup: Super Healthy Recipe

Preparation time: 10-15 mins

Ingredients

- 150 g broccoli
- ½ courgette
- ½ red onion
- 1 C. tablespoon of coconut oil
- 400 ml of water
- 1 bouillon-cube with herbs

Preparation:

1. Cut the red onion and zucchini into small pieces.
2. Then cut the broccoli florets.

3. Heat the coconut oil inside a pan and fry the red onion for about 3 minutes. Then cook the zucchini for 5 minutes.
4. Add the broccoli florets, water, and bouillon cube. Simmer on low heat for 4 minutes.
5. Reduce everything to the blender until you get a creamy soup.
6. This broccoli, zucchini and onion soup can be served immediately or reheated later as you wish. Enjoy your meal!

116. Irish coffee

Person 1

Ingredients

1.5 cl of cane sugar syrup (or 2 pieces of sugar)

2 cl of fresh cream

4 cl of coffee

3 cl of whiskey (bourbon, whiskey)

Preparation

Step 1

Make the "Irish Coffee" recipe directly in the glass.

2nd step

Heat the whiskey with the sugar (at low heat so as not to boil the whiskey) in a saucepan stirring. Prepare a black coffee and pour it over the hot and sweet whiskey, stir slightly. Pour everything into the previously rinsed glass with warm water and coat the surface with lightly beaten cream, it's ready! Savor without delay. To make your cream work better, place it in the freezer for 20 minutes before vigorously whipping it.

Despite some rumors of modern times, an Irish coffee is not supposed to have the three separate floors. Other variants can be made with whipped cream instead of fresh cream, liquid cane sugar instead of powdered sugar or replace the traditional whiskey with whiskey or bourbon, but the original recipe is the one explained above.

Step 3

Serve in a glass type "mug."

Step 4

Add any grated chocolate to the cream.

117. Caramel coffee

Person 1

Ingredients

15 cl of milk

3 cl of caramel syrup

1 dash of cinnamon syrup

1 coffee

Preparation

Step 1

Make the recipe "Coffee Caramel".

2nd step

Make a coffee (espresso). Heat the glass under hot water and pour the caramel syrup into the bottom of the glass. Heat the milk in another container until creamy foam and pour the warm milk gently on the syrup. Pour a few drops of cinnamon syrup and pour the coffee gently over the milk (use a spoon) until you get an extra layer. .

Step 3

Serve in a tumbler type glass.

Step 4

Sprinkle with cinnamon powder.

118. Latte macchiato

Person 1

Ingredients

Coffee

20 cl of milk

Preparation

Step 1

Make the recipe "Latte macchiato" directly in the glass.

2nd step

Beat the milk (preferably whole) with a whisk in a saucepan over the heat to obtain foam on the surface (or using the steam nozzle of your espresso machine).

Pour warm milk into a heat-resistant glass (thick walls), blocking the foam with a spatula.

Add the milk froth on the hot milk.

Finally, gently pour a tight espresso (sweetened according to taste) on the frothed milk.

Since whole milk has a higher density than espresso, the latter will be placed above the milk. .

Step 3

Serve in a tumbler type glass.

Step 4

To serve, you can fill the milk foam with chocolate flakes, liquid caramel, cocoa powder, cinnamon or other spices.

Note

It should not be confused with caffè macchiato.

119. Latte Macchiato Caramel

People 6

Ingredients

1 l of milk

20 cl of coffee

10 cl of caramel syrup

Preparation

Step 1

Make the recipe "Latte Macchiato Caramel" in the pan.

2nd step

Heat the milk and prepare 20 cl of hot black coffee. Divide the milk into 4 large glasses and froth the milk with an emulsifier, electric whisk or steam nozzle on your coffee maker until you have 2 to 3 cm of milk froth.

Pour about 2cl of caramel syrup into each glass and slowly pour 5cl of coffee.

The coffee will come just below the froth of milk, to form 3 layers: the milk at the bottom, the coffee and the milk froth above.

Step 3

Serve in a cup-type glass.

Step 4

Pour a little caramel syrup over the milk froth.

120. Coffee Cream With Caramel Milk Foam

The supreme of pleasure. A creamy cloud of cream of milk and vanilla with toffee flavors.

15 min

Ingredients

Grand Cru Volluto capsule (to prepare 40 ml of Espresso coffee)

100 ml of milk to prepare milk foam

Teaspoon caramel syrup

25 ml / 5 teaspoons of cream (already prepared or homemade according to the method indicated below)

Ingredients for the preparation of 250 ml of homemade cream:

250 ml semi-skimmed milk

2 egg yolks

50 g of white sugar

Half vanilla pod cut lengthwise

Materials

Espresso Cup (80 Ml)

Recipe Spoon Ritual

Preparation

Bring the milk to a boiling point along with half a vanilla pod in a casserole dish

Beat the egg yolks inside a bowl with the sugar

Continue beating the yolks and sugar while adding the milk with the half vanilla pod

Then, put the mixture back in the pan and let it thicken over low heat (do not let the mixture boil to prevent it from cutting)

Check the consistency of the cream with a spoon and, as soon as the cream begins to adhere to the spoon, remove the pan from the heat

Keep stirring the mixture to keep it soft and creamy

Take out the vanilla bean, scrape it with a knife to remove the seeds and put it back in the cream

Prepare a Volluto (25 ml) in an Espresso cup or a small Nespresso recipe glass and add 25 ml / five teaspoons of the homemade cream or ready-made cream

Prepare milk foam with the steam nozzle of your Nespresso machine or the Aeroccino milk frother and add the caramel syrup as soon as the foam begins to form

Cover the coffee cream with the caramel flavored milk foam and serve immediately

121. Hot And Cold Vanilla Espresso With Caramel Foam And Cookies

An exquisite coffee combo with classic flavors of fresh desserts and a delicious cookie accompaniment.

Ingredients

For hot and cold vanilla coffee:

Two capsules of Grand Cru Volluto

A scoop of vanilla ice cream

Three tablespoons of milk foam

Two teaspoons of caramel liquid

For the cookies:

70 g softened butter

70 g of sugar

Teaspoon honey

Egg

100 g flour

a pinch of salt

50 g grated chocolate

For hazelnut caramel:

50 g whole hazelnuts

40 g of sugar

Two tablespoons of water

MATERIALS

Espresso Cup (40 ml)

Oven

Mixer

Preparation

For hot and cold vanilla coffee:

Prepare the milk foam, add the liquid caramel and reserve it

Prepare two coffees in a large cup and pour them into a cold glass

Add the vanilla ice cream ball immediately and cover it with the milk foam

For cookies:

- Preheat oven to 150 °C

Heat sugar and water until caramelized, remove from heat and add crushed hazelnuts

Place the hazelnuts on a sheet of vegetable paper and roast them in the oven for 10 min, moving them occasionally

Put the butter, sugar, salt, honey and egg in a large bowl

Beat it all for a few seconds until you get a smooth mixture

Add caramelized hazelnuts and grated chocolate

Raise the oven temperature to 180 °C

Put small balls of dough on the baking sheet lined with vegetable paper and bake for about 15 min

Let them cool on a rack

122. Espresso With Cottage Cheese, Lime And Brazil Nuts

The sweet lime peel of this creamy mousse with nuts is the perfect balance for the aromatic flavors of the Grand Cru Volluto .

20 min

For 6

Ingredients

One capsule of Grand Cru Volluto or Volluto Decaffeinato

550 g cottage cheese

100 g of sugar

The juice of a lime

Two egg whites

Three jelly sheets or a teaspoon of agar

80 g of Brazil nuts

MATERIALS

A pan: Six molds

Preparation

Roast the Brazil nuts in a pan and mash them finely

Book them

Dip the jelly leaves in cold water to soften them

Grate and squeeze the file

Boil 100 ml of water with sugar and lime juice for 5 minutes

Remove from heat and add the drained gelatin and lime zest

Beat the egg whites and mount them until stiff

Pour three quarters of the lime syrup over the egg whites without stopping to beat and then add the cottage cheese to the mixture

Divide the crushed nuts into the six molds and cover them using a cottage cheese mousse

Pour the remaining lime syrup over and put the molds in the refrigerator for 4 hours

Serve it with a Grand Cru Volluto

123. Coffee with Malice

Ingredients

1 intense espresso coffee sachet

1 splash whiskey

1 splash whole milk or cream

Preparation

3 minutes

You can use dolche gusto machine but if you don't have one you can do it with a good quality soluble coffee loaded. All right; Put the coffee sachet in the coffee maker and select the amount of water to pour.

Activate the hot water until it stops. Have whiskey on hand.

Pour a little squirt of whiskey, heat a little cream or milk and add it to coffee.

Ready, you can add sugar or sweetener if it's your taste. I prefer it as it is. With its bitter touch.

124. Viennese coffee

Delicious!

Ingredients

1 serving

Espresso coffee to your liking.

Whole milk (if you are in full operation bikini... skimmed)

White sugar

Whipped cream

Shavings chocolate

Preparation

5 minutes

Take the coffee capsule. You put it in the machine and let it do its job.

You fill the glass of milk, add your normal dose of sugar and stir.

Decorate with a good tuft of cream and chocolate chips.

As you can see, very, very difficult to do. Having just spent the day.

125. Coffee mousse

Ingredients

6 cups

4 sheets jelly

125 ml espresso coffee

2 tbsps. Baileys

100 gr. sugar

Two egg whites

200 ml 35% mg whipping cream

Preparation

We put to hydrate the gelatin.

We prepare a coffee.

We ride the egg whites with the sugar about to snow.

We semi-cream.

Melt the jello in the hot coffee and add the Baileys.

Add the coffee to tablespoons to the whites mounted.

Add the whipped cream.

We pour the mixture into 6 glasses that we can decorate with sprinkled cocoa powder. In my case I prepared a coffee jelly.

Let cool inside the fridge a few hours and go!

126. Detoxifying milkshake

Also known as weight loss smoothies or green smoothies to clean the body, detox smoothies are easy to prepare and taste delicious – especially when you find ingredients you especially like.

Detox smoothies are powerful to clean the body tool that you can (and should) use every day.

2 people

Time preparation: 10 minutes

Ingredients for 2 people

1 cup of Celery (one head)

2 glass of Spinach

2 glass of Cucumber

1 unit (s) of Limón

2 unit (s) of Apple

1 pinch of fresh ginger

Preparation

Put the ingredients – Celery, Spinach, Cucumber, Limón, Apple, fresh ginger in the blender and then blend till a homogeneous mixture is obtained.

Nutritional composition for 100 grs.

Composition   Amount (gr)   CDR (%)

Kcalories   191.21   10%

Carbohydrates   29.52   9.5%

Proteins   7.32   15.3%

127. Green pineapple smoothie

Considering how challenging it is to eat enough vegetables in your diet, drinking the green smoothie makes you believe like you have accomplished a health goal for the day.

1 person

Time preparation: 5 minutes

Ingredients for 1 person

50 grams of Chard

1 unit (s) of Apple

200 grams of Pineapple

1 teaspoon of Flax seeds

Preparation

Add Chard, Apple, Pineapple, Flax seeds all to the glass of the blender with a little water and grind well.

Nutritional composition for 100 grs.

Composition	Amount (gr)	CDR (%)
Kcalories	251.16	13.1%
Carbohydrates	46.44	14.9%
Proteins	3.51	7.3%

128. Chile Campana Smoothie

Ingredients

One medium banana, peeled fresh or frozen

1 can (8 ounces) pineapple, drained

1/2 cup of red bell pepper, cored and diced (about 1 small bell pepper)

2 cups of frozen mixed berries

1 cup of water

Preparation:

Combine all ingredients inside a blender or food processor.

Blend thoroughly until lump free.

Serve immediately.

Refrigerate or freeze what is within the next 2 hours.

Notes

For a sweeter smoothie, reserve and add canned pineapple juice. Use less water if you are adding juice.

Use any combination of berries.

129. Pumpkin Smoothie in a Glass

Ingredients

2/3 cup of yogurt vanilla flavored, low fat or one container (6 ounces)

1/4 cup of pumpkin canned

2 teaspoons of brown sugar

1/4 teaspoon of cinnamon

1/8 teaspoon of nutmeg (optional)

Preparation

Stir all the ingredients together inside a bowl. Serve.

Refrigerate what about within the next 2 hours.

Notes

Put granola or cereal chips on top for an extra crispy smoothie.

You can freeze canned squash that you can use later on main dishes, soups, chili or cooked food.

130. Berry and Beet Smoothie

Ingredients

1 cup of pineapple juice

1 cup of low-fat or fat-free vanilla yogurt

1 cup of fresh or frozen strawberries

1/2 cup of fresh or frozen blueberries

1/2 cup of beet canned sliced, drained

Preparation

Combine all ingredients in a blender.

Mix until smooth.

Serve immediately.

Refrigerate or freeze what is left over during the next 2 hours.

Notes

For a thicker smoothie, use frozen fruit instead of fresh fruit.

Use plain yogurt and ½ teaspoon of vanilla.

Add a banana.

131. Pumpkin Spread Cream

Ingredients

1 can (15 ounces) pumpkin (about 1 ¾ cups cooked pumpkin)

1 cup of low-fat ricotta cheese or plain yogurt or low-fat cream cheese

3/4 cup of sugar

1 1/2 teaspoon of cinnamon

1/2 teaspoon of nutmeg

Preparation

In a large bowl, combine pumpkin, ricotta or yogurt, sugar, cinnamon and nutmeg. Stir until the mixture is completely smooth.

Refrigerate what about within the next 2 hours.

Notes

Serve with apple wedges, bananas or grapes.

For a softer texture, use a hand blender or food processor to mix the ingredients.

132. Chilling raspberry

Ingredients

1 cup of raspberries

two Bananas

1/2 cup of yogurt natural, low fat

1/4 cup of milk 1% or nonfat

1 tsp. of sugar

Preparation

Put all the ingredients in the blender. Blend until lump free.

Divide the mixture between 4 small containers.

Freeze for about 2 hours or so. Enjoy as if it were snow or ice cream!

Freeze or refrigerate what is within the next 2 hours.

Notes

Do not have a blender? Crush the fruits well with a fork.

Make ice popsicles! Serve the mixture with a spoon in small paper cups or molds to make ice lollipops. Add a wooden stick for crafts. Freeze until firm so that the stick does not come out.

133. Popeye's Powerful Smoothie

Ingredients

1 cup of orange juice

1/2 cup of pineapple juice

1/2 cup of natural-flavored or vanilla yogurt, "low fat or 1 recipient

One Banana, peeled and sliced

2 cups of spinach leaves fresh

Crushed ice

Preparation

Combine all ingredients in a blender.

Mix well until smooth.

Serve immediately.

Refrigerate what is inside in the next 2 hours.

Notes

For a thicker smoothie, use frozen fruit.

Use any type of juice.

134. Smoothie ananas plant infusion

This is a refreshing and delicious drink. Pineapple is a bromeliad that helps drain cellulite and is rich in vitamin c. You can add the infusion of your choice.

Preparation time: 10 minutes

Servings 2 people

Ingredients

1/2 fresh pineapple
250 ml infusion (plant of your choice)
1 hypertonic quinton water
1/2 lemon (juice)

Preparation

1. Peel a fresh pineapple
2. Cut it in half to remove the stick (or heart) more efficiently by turning with a thin knife
3. Take one half of pineapple and cut into pieces to help the blender
4. Once mixed, add the lemon juice
5. Take a brew that has been kept cool (or prepare one in advance and let cool) (the plant is your choice; you can also make tea). Add the infusion to the mousse
6. Blend a blender to mix the two liquids that are

superimposed because the pineapple is sparkling is lighter
7. Add hypertonic quinton water that will give this smoothie a little pep
8. Mix and serve in glasses
9. Two very cold beverages are obtained (if the ingredients are taken out of the refrigerator). Otherwise, leave 1 hour in the fridge before serving or add some ice cubes
10. This drink is very delicious with the foam that gives an even more pleasant sensation;

Nutrition facts

Calories 50   % daily value
Total fat 0.1 g   0%
Saturated fat 0 g   0%
Polyunsaturated fat 0 g
Monounsaturated fat 0 g
Cholesterol 0 mg   0%
Sodium 1 mg   0%
Potassium 109 mg   3%
Total carbohydrate 13 g   4%
Dietary fiber 1.4 g   5%
Sugar 10 g
Protein 0.5 g   1%

135. Lemon cream

For this lemon cream we need:

Ingredients:

230 gr of sugar

25 cl of water

Two egg whites

One little bit of lemon zest

Lemon juice (1 lemon)

Preparation:

In a bit of cactus, we are going to put the water, the sugar, the juice, and the lemon zest.

We mix it well and put it in the blender, where we will add the whites that we have assembled beforehand. We beat until we have a creamy texture.

136. Grouper in green sauce

A soft and delicious low-calorie fish easy to prepare and serve in green tomatillo sauce

Yield: 2 servings

Ingredients

- 2 grouper fillets
- Salt and pepper
- 1 tablespoon of olive oil

For the sauce:

- 2 tomatillos, without the peel
- ¼ cup of pumpkin seeds
- ½ cup of green paprika, without seeds or veins
- ½ cup of coriander leaves only
- ½ of a jalapeño, without seeds or veins
- ½ cup of parsley leaves only
- ½ teaspoon fresh thyme
- 3 garlic cloves
- ¼ cup of fish stock
- 1 pinch of salt

Preparation:

1. In a medium saucepan with water at the time, add the tomatillos and boil 1 minute. Stir and place in the blender.
2. In a medium skillet, add the seeds and toast on low, medium heat for 1 to 2 minutes or until golden brown. Remove and place in the blender.
3. Pour the rest of the ingredients. Blend well.

4. Pour out the sauce into the pan and then cook over medium heat for 1 minute.
5. Dry the fish fillets with the paper towel and salt and pepper to taste.
6. In another wide pan, add the olive oil and let it heat over medium-high heat.
7. Place the steaks and let them brown, 3 to 4 minutes on each side. Serve with the sauce.

137. Pumpkin and apple soup

Ingredients

- 450 grams (1 lb.) Pumpkin
- 1 granny smith apple cored, and quartered
- One medium onion cut
- Two cloves garlic
- One tablespoon of olive oil

- Salt
- ¼ teaspoon of cayenne more to taste
- 300 ml (1¼ cup) of vegetable stock
- Freshly ground black pepper to add taste

Garnish:
- Pomegranate arils
- Some pumpkin seeds
- Fresh parsley finely chopped

Preparation

1. Preheat the oven about 200 degrees c (or 392 degrees f). Line a large baking sheet with a parchment paper.
2. Cut the pumpkin half lengthways and scoop out seeds.
3. Slice each pumpkin half in half to make quarters and place, cut-side up, on a baking tray, along with the onions.
4. Drizzle with olive oil and then sprinkle some salt.
5. Bake for about 20 minutes, then add the garlic and apple, flip the pumpkin cut side down and then roast for another for 20 minutes, or until the flesh is soft.
6. Take one spoon to scoop out the flesh of the pumpkin and transfer to a high-speed blender with

the apple, onion, garlic (remove the skins), cayenne, and vegetable stock.
7. Blend on high for almost 2 minutes, or until silky smooth.
8. If too thick, add vegetable stock to thin it out and blend over. Taste and adjust the seasonings.
9. Serve, ladle soup into a bowl, and with pomegranate arils, pumpkin seeds, fresh parsley and freshly ground black pepper.
10. Then serve.
11. Refrigerate leftovers inside an airtight container for 4 days,

138. Double melon mojito

Use any melon you have on hand. You can also choose to use a rum flavored with melon.

Makes 1 a glass of 10 ounces.

Ingredients

- 6 to 10 fresh mint leaves, plus 1 sprig to decorate
- 1 small file, cut in half, plus a slice to decorate
- ¼ cup melon in pieces (use any type, such as cantaloupe, chinese melon or watermelon), plus some small pieces to garnish
- 2 tablespoons of simple stevia syrup or simple sugar syrup
- 1 line (1½ ounces) of white rum or rum flavored with melon
- 1 cup of ice
- ½ cup of soda water

Preparation

1. Place the mint leaves in a strong glass.

2. Squeeze the lime halves over the mint. Use a crusher to crush the mint and extract the aromatic oils lightly.

3. Add the melon and lightly squeeze it with the crusher.

4. Pour the syrup and rum into the glass, stirring. Stretch the preparation, if you prefer.

5. Add ice and soda water. Stir

6. Dress the glass with the sprig of mint, the slice of the lime and the small pieces of melon, and let the melon pieces float in the drink.

139. Basil and blackberry mojito

This recipe replaces the mint with basil. It is also great if it is made with strawberries.

Makes 1 a glass of 10 ounces.

Ingredients

- 6 to 10 leaves of fresh basil, plus a sprig to decorate
- 1 small file, cut in half, plus a slice to decorate
- ¼ cup of blackberries, plus a few extras to garnish
- 2 tablespoons of simple stevia syrup or simple sugar syrup
- 1 line (1½ ounces) of white rum
- 1 cup of ice
- ½ cup of soda water

Preparation

1. Place the mint leaves in a strong glass.

2. Squeeze the lime halves over the mint. Use a crusher to crush the mint lightly and then extract the aromatic oils.

3. Add the blackberries and squash them lightly with the crusher until they release their juice.

4. Pour the syrup and rum into the glass, stirring. Stretch the preparation, if you prefer.

5. Add ice and soda water. Stir

6. Garnish the glass with the sprig of basil, the slice of lime and the extra blackberries, and let the blackberries float in the drink.

140. Tart apple and carrots soup

Ingredients

- 800 g carrots
- 2 golden apples
- 1 onion
- 1.5 liters of water
- 1 cubic broth of vegetables preferably
- Ginger
- Salt pepper

Preparation

1. Wash and peel the carrots and apples, cut into small pieces.
2. Cut the onion and sweat it in a pan with oil.
3. Add carrots and apples.
4. In a saucepan, melt the cubed vegetable broth in 1.5 liters of water.
5. Cover the vegetables with the broth.
6. Season and boil for 30 minutes.
7. Mix everything together.

141. Black bean and avocado soup

Ingredients

Servings: 10

- 1 can (540 ml) of black beans, well drained
- 1 can (398 ml) corn kernels, drained
- 4 roma tomatoes, seeded and chopped
- 1 red pepper, diced
- 1 jalapeno pepper, chopped
- 1/3 cup chopped fresh cilantro
- 1/4 cup red onion
- 1/4 cup fresh lime juice
- 2 tbsp. Red wine vinegar
- 1 c. Salt
- 1/2 c. Pepper
- 2 lawyers, diced

Preparations

Combine all ingredients except avocados inside a big bowl and mix. Add the avocados and mix gently. Cover with plastic wrap (directly on the salsa) and refrigerate at least 2 hours before serving.

142. Cream of pear and arugula

Quantity: 2 Persians

Preparation: 20 minutes

Cooling: 15-20 minutes

Ingredients:

Half a liter of water

4 pears blanquillos with leather, at its point of maturation

1 bowl of arugula

2 tablespoons of fresh aromatic herbs

The juice of 1 small lemon

Sea salt or herbal salt

1 pinch of ground black pepper

Extra virgin olive oil

Edible flowers to decorate

Preparation:

1. Grind whole the ingredients in the blender jar, except extra virgin olive oil and flowers, until a creamy and

homogeneous texture is obtained. If necessary, rectify water, salt, and pepper.

2. Refrigerate until ready to serve and, once in the bowl, decorate with the flowers and a thread of olive oil. If you do not have flowers, you can use chopped almonds, some rocket leaves or sesame seeds.

3. If you do not have a bowl of arugula you can also use other green leaves such as spinach, lamb's lettuce, watercress, mustard greens, etc. with the aromatic herbs, the same: you can make with parsley, dill, chives, basil, cilantro or mint. To know more: The pear is a fruit with satiating effect for its fiber content: it is fantastic for people who want to lose weight and are doing a diet to lose weight. Also, it is a fruit with anti-inflammatory action, helps us maintain a regular intestinal transit and combat constipation, and has a very beneficial effect on our microbiota or intestinal flora. Choose it whenever you can from organic farming.

Nutritional Information

Calories   197.1

Total Fat 12.1 g

Saturated Fat   3.2 g

Polyunsaturated Fat   3.5 g

Monounsaturated Fat 4.1 g

Cholesterol	10.0 mg

Sodium	181.2 mg

Potassium	149.7 mg

Total Carbohydrate	21.3 g

Dietary Fiber	3.0 g

Sugars	15.9 g

Protein	3.5 g

143. Soup 'green

Quantity: 1 person

Preparation: 15 minutes

Refrigeration: 15 minutes (optional)

Ingredients:

Water in sufficient quantity to achieve the desired texture

1 green apple with skin

1 slice of fresh peeled ginger

Half lemon or 1 lime without skin, the white part without seeds

Half cucumber with skin

Half bowl of leaves with fresh spinach

1 bunch of basil or fresh cilantro

1 branch of wireless celery, including tender green leaves

Preparation:

1. Wash and chop all the ingredients. Insert them into the glass of blender and crush.

2. Add the water and crush again until you get a homogeneous texture. If necessary, rectify water.

3. Take the soup as a snack at any time of the day to purify the body and keep cravings at bay. To know more: This cold soup is quick to prepare and has great benefits for the body. Perhaps the best-known property of the apple is its intestinal regulatory action. If we eat it raw and with skin, it is useful to treat constipation, since this way we take advantage of its richness in insoluble fiber present in the skin, which stimulates the intestinal activity and helps to keep the intestinal muscles in shape. Also, green apples are one of the largest sources of flavonoids. These antioxidant compounds can stop the action of free radicals on the cells of the body. Eating raw fruits and vegetables is the healthiest option.

Nutritional Information

Calories 330

Fat 12 g 18 %

Saturated 1.7 g

+ Trans 0 g 8 %

Cholesterol 90 mg

Sodium 240 mg 10 %

Carbohydrate 20 g 6 %

Fibre 5 g 22 %

Sugars 4 g

Net Carbs 15 g

Protein 38 g

Vitamin A 4 %

Vitamin C 45 %

Calcium 10 %

Iron 15 %

144. Greek chicken stew with slow cooker

Prep 25 min

Total 9 hr 40 min

Portions 6

Enhanced flavors of the Aegean Sea, such as cinnamon and lemon zest, turn this slow cooker chicken into a quick-flavored, fast-cooking stew with canned tomatoes and frozen onions.

Ingredients

- 2 t. (500 mL) mini-carrots, cut in half lengthwise if large
- 3 onions, quartered
- 6 chicken legs with bone, without skin
- 1 C. (5 mL) ground cinnamon
- 1/2 c. (2 mL) salt
- 1/2 c. (2 mL) pepper
- 2 garlic cloves, finely chopped
- 1 can (28 oz / 796 mL) diced tomatoes, not drained
- 1/3 t. (75 mL) tomato paste
- 2 tbsp. (10 mL) grated lemon rind
- 1/2 c. (2 mL) dried oregano leaves
- 1/4 t. (50 mL) chopped parsley

Preparation

1. Spray 4 to the 5-quart crockpot with cooking spray. Place the carrots and onions in the slow cooker. Place the chicken legs on the vegetables. Sprinkle with cinnamon, salt, pepper, and garlic; pour the tomatoes on the whole. Cover and then cook it on low heat for 7 to 9 hours or until vegetables are tender and chicken is easy to peel with a fork.
2. Remove the chicken with a dripping spoon and cover to keep warm. Stir in the tomato paste, lemon zest and oregano in the slow cooker broth. Cover; cook 15 minutes or until everything is thick and hot. In the meantime, discard the bones from the chicken. Return the chicken to the slow cooker, stirring and cutting the larger pieces.
3. To serve, spoon stew within shallow bowls and garnish with parsley.

Nutritional value

Serving: 6 servings

- calories200
- Fat6
- Saturated fatty acids2 Trans fat0
- Cholesterol45 Sodium580 Total carbohydrates20
- Dietary fiber5 sugars10
- Protein17

145. Southwestern Chicken Chili Cooked In Slow Cooker

Prep 20 min

Total 8 hr 20 min

Servings 8

Warm up your winter evenings with this spicy soup that only takes 20 minutes to cook.

Ingredients

- 1 t. (250 mL) onions, chopped
- 1 t. (250 mL) chopped green pepper
- 1 C. 5 mL ground cumin
- 1/2 c. (2 mL) salt
- 1/4 lb. (625 g) boneless skinless chicken thighs, cut into 1 inch (2.5 cm) pieces
- 1 bowl (440 mL) Old El Paso * Picante sauce medium (about 2 t.)
- 1 can (540 mL / 19 fl. Oz.) Of Pinto beans or kidney beans, drained
- 1 can (398 mL / 14 fl. Oz.) Diced tomatoes, drained

- Green onion, sliced, if desired
- 3 cloves of garlic, minced
- 3 c. (45 mL) cornmeal
- 2 tbsp. (25 mL) chili powder
- 3 c. (15 mL) dried oregano leaves

Preparation

1. In a slow cooker with 3 to 4 qt (3 to 4 L) capacity, combine the onions, pepper and garlic.
2. In a large bowl, combine cornmeal, chili powder, oregano, cumin and salt. Stir in the chicken; stir to coat. Add the chicken mixture and all remaining seasonings to the vegetables in the slow cooker. Gently stir Picante sauce, beans and tomatoes.
3. Cover; then cook over low heat for 6 to 8 hours. Sprinkle with green onions

Sirtfood Snacks

146. Sand Cheese And Apple Pie

INGREDIENTS

- Cinnamon – pinch
- Cottage cheese - 500 g
- An Apple - 1 kg
- Baking powder - 1 teaspoon
- Margarine - 200 g
- Sugar - 1.5 cups
- Wheat flour - 2 cups
- Sour cream - 100 g
- Chicken egg - 4 pieces

PREPARATION

7. For the test, grind 3 yolks (we carefully separate them with proteins) with 0.5 cups of sugar, then grind with softened (not melted) margarine (butter), then introduce the flour, baking powder, knead a rather thick dough with your hands, finally mix in roll sour cream into a bowl, cover and refrigerate for at least half an hour while the filling is being prepared and the oven is preheated

8. Rub the cottage cheese, mix with 1/3 cup sugar and 1 yolk (add the protein from the egg to the remaining three)
9. Peel the apples and seeds, cut into thin slices (until the dough is rolled out, it is better to sprinkle them with lemon juice or diluted citric acid so that they do not darken, but you can cut them already when the cake is ready to be planted in the oven).
10. Roll out the dough thin enough on a rather large baking sheet, making sides along the edges (so that the curd does not drip). We spread evenly the curd filling, beautifully lay the apple slices on it, and sprinkle with cinnamon. We put the oven preheated to 200 degrees for 30-40 minutes.
11. While the cake is baking, beat the whites with the remaining sugar in a thick foam.
12. Take out the slightly baked cake and lay the protein foam over the apples evenly, level it and put it in the hot oven again. When in a few minutes the squirrels grab a light brown crust - the cake is ready!!!

147. COTTAGE CHEESE "STRAWBERRIES WITH CREAM"

INGREDIENTS

- Fat cottage cheese-800 gr.
- Semolina-5 tbsp.
- Eggs - 3-4 pcs.
- Salt-1/2 tsp
- Sugar 1/2 tbsp. (adjust to your liking)
- Vanilla
- Dried fruits (raisins or whatever you like. I have a citrus flavor, candied pamello)

For cream and filling:

- Fresh strawberries_200-300 gr.
- Fat cream (sour cream) -3-4 tablespoons
- Sugar.

PREPARATION

6. Wipe the cottage cheese through a fine sieve.
7. Blatter the eggs with sugar, salt and vanilla, add the egg mixture to the curd, put the semolina, sliced candied fruit, mix and put into the mold, pre-greased it with vegetable oil and sprinkled with cereal.

8. Cut the strawberries into plates; lay them tightly on the curd dough.
9. Separately, prepare the cream, whip the sour cream or cream with sugar and apply the cream on the strawberries.
10. Bake the manna until cooked, but do not overdo it in the oven.

148. WINTER MULLED WINE

INGREDIENT

- Water - 1.5 cups
- Dry red wine - 1.5 cups
- Cinnamon sticks - 2 pieces
- Clove - 3 pieces
- Grated lemon zest – pinch
- Oranges - 1 piece
- Honey - 6 tablespoons
- Sugar - 2 tablespoons
- Anise (star anise) - 3 pieces
- Ground ginger - on the tip of a knife
- Black tea – taste

PREPARATION

1. Pour water into a pot and bring to a boil.

2. Throw tea and spices.

3. Pour the wine and toss the sliced orange.

4. Add sugar and honey.

5. Cook for 6 minutes without boiling.

149. BANANA CRUMBLE

INGREDIENTS

- Butter - 50 g
- Sugar - 2 tbsp.
- Wheat flour - 3 tbsp. (with a slide)
- Walnut Kernels - 30 g
- Banana - 2 pcs.

PREPARATION

9. Combine cold butter with sugar and flour.
10. Stir with a quick motion with a fork (or rub with your hands) until crumbs form.
11. Chop walnuts with a knife into medium pieces and add to the sand mass. Mix
12. Peel and slice the bananas into small pieces.
13. Put the bananas in a suitable shape. For the preparation of crumble, you can take portioned molds or one large one.
14. On top of the bananas, evenly distribute all the chips.
15. Send the dessert form to the oven preheated to 180 degrees. Bake for 20-25 minutes, until golden brown.
16. Delicious banana crumble can be served.

150. STRAWBERRY CAKE "CLOUD"

INGREDIENTS

- Cookies - 150 g
- Coconut Chips - 0.5 cups
- Butter - 100 g
- Ground cinnamon - 0.5-1 tsp
- Egg white - 2 pcs.
- Sugar - 1 cup or slightly less (to taste)
- Strawberry - 250 g
- Lemon juice - 1 tbsp.
- Vanilla or vanilla sugar to taste

Additionally:

- Cardamom - 4-6 boxes

PREPARATION

12. Grind cookies with a blender or rolling pin.
13. Combine chopped cookies and coconut. Add cinnamon, melted butter and mix well.
14. Cover the bottom of the detachable shape with parchment paper.

15. Put the cookie mixture into the mold. Flatten by pressing with a spoon or fingers. The base should not be thick; otherwise, when it hardens in the freezer, to cut it, you will have to try. It is enough that it only covers the bottom of the form with a continuous even thin layer.
16. Place the cake pan in the refrigerator or freezer to cool.
17. Now let's prepare the very "cloud". Take a large bowl - the mixture will greatly increase in volume. Combine egg whites, sugar, strawberries, lemon juice and vanilla. If possible, add some ground cardamom - an incredibly tasty combination.
18. Beat everything first until smooth, and then continue to whisk until the mixture has tripled in volume. Use room temperature proteins to speed up the process.
    Rub a drop of protein mass with your fingertips, sugar grains should not be felt.
19. Put the protein mixture on the cooled cake and smooth.
20. Place in the freezer for 4 hours. While the cake is cooling, in addition to it, you can make quick strawberry sauce.
21. Strawberry Cake "Cloud" is ready! Decorate the finished cake as desired. Store the cake in the

freezer. In a sealed container, the cake can be stored for up to 1 month.
22. Cut the cake, after dipping the blade of the knife in hot water for a few seconds. In the freezer, the cake cools and hardens. But it will become airy and tender, like a cloud, after only a few minutes at room temperature.

Are Sirtfoods The New Superfoods?

There is no doubt that sirtfoods are good for the body. The benefits of almost all of them are confirmed by scientific research. For example, consuming a moderate amount of dark chocolate with a high cocoa content can reduce the risk of heart disease and assist fight inflammation.

Green tea reduces the risk of stroke and diabetes and helps lower blood pressure. Turmeric has anti-inflammatory properties, has a beneficial effect on the body as a whole, and protects against many chronic diseases. At the same time, evidence for the health benefits of increasing sirtuin levels is less obvious. So far, only animal studies and cell cultures have shown interesting results.

For example, it was found that an increase in sirtuin levels leads to an increase in life expectancy in yeast, worms, and mice. Also, during fasting or calorie restriction, sirtuins help the body burn more fat and improve insulin sensitivity.

Is It Healthy and Sustainable

Sirtfoods are healthy and healthy foods that undoubtedly can have a positive effect on health due to their antioxidant and anti-inflammatory properties. However, eating only a handful of very healthy foods cannot satisfy all the needs of the body. The Sirtfood diet is overly restrictive and does not provide clear, unique health benefits compared to other types of diets.

Also, this diet is prescribed to drink up to three glasses of juice per day. Although this juice can be a good source of vitamins and minerals, it contains almost no healthy fiber needed by the body. In addition, the diet is so limited in calories and food choices that it is highly likely to lead to a deficiency of protein, vitamins, and minerals, especially at the first stage.

Due to its low-calorie content and limited choice of food, this diet can be difficult to follow for all three weeks. Adding here the high costs of buying a juicer, books, and some rare and expensive ingredients, as well as spending time preparing special dishes and juice, the diet becomes completely unfeasible for many people.

Safety and Side Effects

Although the first stage of the Sirtfood diet contains very few calories and is an inadequate diet, given the short duration of the diet, it is unlikely to be dangerous for an average healthy adult. However, in people with diabetes, calorie restriction, and eating large amounts of juice during the first few days can cause dangerous spikes in blood sugar levels.

Also, because of the low-calorie content and low fiber content in your diet, you are likely to feel severe hunger for all three weeks. During the first phase, you may even encounter side effects such as increased fatigue and irritability.

Conclusion

Objectively speaking, sirtfood was developed not only and not so much as, in fact, a diet for weight loss, but as an effective antiage program. Moreover, acting in a short time. According to the plan, the express program should increase the "productivity" of the body - its energy reserves, resistance to stress and aging processes. Initially, sirtfood food was recommended for football players and participants in rowing regattas. And later it turned out that he has a bonus that is relevant for a wider public: the ability to lose weight and stop the feeling of hunger.

Wine, dark chocolate and all-all-all

So, what foods make up the sirtfood diet? Oddly enough, with such a diet you can even have sweets . Specifically, dark chocolate (at least 85%) and red wine, rich in polyphenols.

MEDITERRANEAN DIET COOKBOOK FOR BEGINNERS

The Ultimate Quick and Easy Guide on How to Effectively Lose Weight, Prevent Heart Disease with MOUTHWATERING RECIPES to INCREASE ENERGY AND HEAL THE BODY FOR LIFELONG HEALTH

G.S. Van Leeuwen

© COPYRIGHT 2020 ALL RIGHTS RESERVED. G.S. VAN LEEUWEN

THIS DOCUMENT IS GEARED TOWARDS PROVIDING EXACT AND RELIABLE INFORMATION WITH REGARD TO THE TOPIC AND ISSUE COVERED. THE PUBLICATION IS SOLD WITH THE IDEA THAT THE PUBLISHER IS NOT REQUIRED TO RENDER ACCOUNTING, OFFICIALLY PERMITTED, OR OTHERWISE QUALIFIED SERVICES. IF ADVICE IS NECESSARY, LEGAL OR PROFESSIONAL, A PRACTICED INDIVIDUAL IN THE PROFESSION SHOULD BE ORDERED. FROM A DECLARATION OF PRINCIPLES WHICH WAS ACCEPTED AND APPROVED EQUALLY BY A COMMITTEE OF THE AMERICAN BAR ASSOCIATION AND A COMMITTEE OF PUBLISHERS AND ASSOCIATIONS.IN NO WAY IS IT LEGAL TO REPRODUCE, DUPLICATE, OR TRANSMIT ANY PART OF THIS DOCUMENT IN EITHER ELECTRONIC MEANS OR IN PRINTED FORMAT. RECORDING OF THIS PUBLICATION IS STRICTLY PROHIBITED, AND ANY STORAGE OF THIS DOCUMENT IS NOT ALLOWED UNLESS WITH WRITTEN PERMISSION FROM THE PUBLISHER. ALL RIGHTS RESERVED.THE INFORMATION PROVIDED HEREIN IS STATED TO BE TRUTHFUL AND CONSISTENT, IN THAT ANY LIABILITY, IN TERMS OF INATTENTION OR OTHERWISE, BY ANY USAGE OR ABUSE OF ANY POLICIES, PROCESSES, OR DIRECTIONS CONTAINED WITHIN IS THE SOLITARY AND UTTER RESPONSIBILITY OF THE RECIPIENT READER. UNDER NO CIRCUMSTANCES WILL ANY LEGAL RESPONSIBILITY OR BLAME BE HELD AGAINST THE PUBLISHER FOR ANY REPARATION, DAMAGES, OR MONETARY LOSS DUE TO THE INFORMATION HEREIN, EITHER DIRECTLY OR INDIRECTLY.

INTRODUCTION

Healthy living is a treasured luxury that doesn't come by itself. You have to schedule it. Nutrition plays a crucial role in supplying the body with essential nutrients for growth and development. While some foods are considered healthy and in large quantities are required, others may be excluded from a daily diet. So works a Mediterranean diet plan.

The most common type of healthy diet is the Mediterranean diet. Studies have proved that people in the Mediterranean region can attribute the secret of healthy living to their balanced diet and active lifestyles. Researches have also shown that not only does this diet alleviate chronic heart disease, it also increases life expectancy.

Today's habits show that most people prefer to eat fried, frozen, or tinned foods that contain saturated fats and sugar. Lifestyles often suggest that most people don't take the time to exercise. As a result, with an increased chance of heart disease, diabetes and cancers, many people are obese and unhealthy.

The Mediterranean diet plan does not reduce the food types that one eats. The diet advises wise choices regarding food. For starters, instead of tinned and frozen food, one should eat fresh fruit and vegetables.

The food plan is based on the pyramid Mediterranean diet. According to him, cereals, grains, pasta, vegetables, legumes, beans, fruit, and nuts are food products to be included in a daily diet. These nutritious goods are a rich source of carbohydrates, fabrics, vitamins, minerals, and proteins. The recommended milk, yogurt and cheese consumption, low to moderate, reduce excessive intake of saturated fats. Animal meat such as chicken and eggs shall be consumed regularly and red meat, several times a month. Fish is considered a better choice, since it is high in nutritional value.

Olive oil provides good fat, which is responsible for reducing blood cholesterol levels and maintaining a healthy heart. All these recommendations are in line with a regular diet recommendation in the Mediterranean diet plan. A balanced dietary intake through an active physical life. This is not to say that people did not find time to rest in the Mediterranean area. They also used the time to relax and socialize after each meal, unwittingly giving time for proper digestion and good health.

CHAPTER ONE
Understanding the Mediterranean diet

The Mediterranean diet is one of the propagated diets, but that many people still don't know. It is usually a very simple diet and one of the most suitable, since it involves small risks to health.

Your idea is very simple and clear, and you always get interesting results done in a correct and specified way. It is from this transition that you will achieve your goal of a healthy weight loss, always with a consistent schedule.

Let's bring about what it treats for those who don't know about this diet, and also other factors that may enhance its action. From this, you can change your reality in favor of a type of diet that is very appropriate even for those who don't seek weight loss themselves.

The Mediterranean diet includes a large number of fruits, vegetables, beans, nuts, seeds, bread and other cereals. In the Mediterranean diet, fruits and vegetables are usually grown locally. Raw or minimally processed fruits and vegetables are often consumed. Fruit and vegetables contain many essential vitamins and minerals as well as antioxidants which are essential for good health.

The primary source of fat for the Mediterranean Diet is the use of monounsaturated fat. Olive oil is monounsaturated fat which is a rich antioxidant source like vitamin E. Olive oil is used as an alternative to butter, margarine and other fats. Butter and cream in fact are used only on special occasions. In the Mediterranean diet, olive oil is used for cooking tomato sauces, vegetable dishes, salads, and frying fish.

What is the Mediterranean diet

The Mediterranean diet is a set of human-related skills, knowledge, practices and traditions, ranging from land to table, covering crops, crops and fishing, as well as preserving, processing and preparing food and, in particular, its consumption.

This diet's nutritional model has remained constant over time and space, with the main ingredients being olive oil, cereals, fresh or dried fruits and vegetables, a moderate proportion of meat, fish and dairy products, abundant condiments and wine or infusions accompanying their consumption at the table, always respecting the beliefs of each community.

The Mediterranean diet-whose name derives from the Greek word regular, which means the way of life-comprises not only food, as it is a cultural element that promotes social interaction, verifying that traditional meals are a cornerstone of customs celebrations and festive events. Additionally, the Mediterranean diet gave rise to a large body of knowledge, poems, choruses, tales and legends.

One of the few diets that affect the health of those who adopt it is the Mediterranean diet. As you'll know a little later, this isn't even a diet, but rather a lifestyle that can be practiced for life.

When we think about diets, thoughts about poverty, hunger and the intake of tasteless foods always come to mind. That should not however be the case. Diet is a diet in which we choose to focus on eating other foods while limiting or reducing the consumption of others. Dieting is a diet that can aim for weight loss as well as weight gain. In addition to reducing weight, the diet may also aim to improve the symptoms of a variety of medical conditions that are closely related to food. These include, for example, type 2 diabetes, high cholesterol, high blood pressure, metabolic syndrome and even cancer.

When we want to follow a particular diet or diet to improve our health, the changes we make must be long-term. The Mediterranean Diet is one long-term diet. Not even a diet; it is a diet that we choose to follow for a long time or for life.

History of the Mediterranean diet

In recent years, there has been increasing concern for their health among men and women in different countries around the world. Many men and women often paid more attention to their meals, as many people were more concerned with their general health. Both men and women basically make dietary choices to boost their overall health and wellbeing.

A significant number of these men and women became interested in the Mediterranean diet as people became more aware of their health and nutrition. Yes, if you're a person who appreciates the food-health relationship, you may have a keen interest in the history of the Mediterranean diet.

Before you can fully understand what the Mediterranean diet is all about, you have to be mindful that it is more of a philosophy than a single eating regimen. There is in fact no Mediterranean diet popular to all Mediterranean countries around the world. Instead, the "Mediterranean Diet" consists of the foods that people consume together in the different nations of the region.

The Origins of the Mediterranean Diet

The concept of a Mediterranean diet derives from the eating habits and patterns of the people who populate Italy, Greece, Spain, France, Tunisia, Lebanon and Morocco. As a result, the Mediterranean diet also includes a huge variety of delicious foods. In reality, if a person chooses to embrace the Mediterranean dining scheme definition, or if a person chooses to pursue a Mediterranean diet system, he or she will have the ability to enjoy a vast range of scrumptious food.

The diet of the peoples who populated the Mediterranean Sea regions has, in fact, remained almost unchanged for well over a thousand years. The region's history is full of examples of men and women living longer than similarly situated people consuming alternate diets. Through the centuries, people in the Mediterranean Sea region have enjoyed longer lives at the same historical epoch than people in other parts of the world.

Foods and beverages which are indigenous to the geographic landmass surrounding the Mediterranean Sea are at the heart of the Mediterranean diet. In short, the development of the Mediterranean diet and dining pattern developed initially by providential. The region's people ate those foods naturally and understandably, and drank those beverages that were readily available in and around their homes.

Historical elements of the Mediterranean diet scheme

As already mentioned, the diet of the Mediterranean Sea region's peoples has remained essentially unchanged over the centuries. The Mediterranean diet is made up of a plethora of healthy food items including:

- Fresh fruit
- Fresh vegetables
- Low-fat nuts
- Whole grains
- Monounsaturated fat

The Mediterranean diet used by people for generation after generation, in a similar vein, excludes or limits certain food items that have been deemed harmful in recent scientific studies. These food items are less than desirable and include:

- Saturated fats
- Red and fatty meat
- Rich dairy products
- Fatty fish

The so-called Mediterranean diet is the historical evolution of the Mediterranean Sea basin through generations of cultures and civilizations.

Man learns to grow certain plant species 10,000 years ago, and domesticates certain animals, ceases to be nomadic and creates stable population settlements, usually in areas with good climate and water.

Nutrition is already expressed in many texts in the ancient civilizations of Babylon and Egypt. We make observations about foods that should or should not be eaten and one of them is also forbidden.

The basin of the Mediterranean is a crossroads of nations, languages, cultures, and religions. With various eating practices, diets, fasts, ritual meals, etc. Driven by Christianity, Judaism, and Islam.

The Greeks, Punics, and Romans entered the Mediterranean with wheat, vineyards, and olive trees.

The Germans the rice, citrus, eggplant and dried pasta Muslims butter.

American basic foods were imported from America, such as tomatoes, peppers, and potatoes.

Based on a natural balance of fish and vegetable meats, with plenty of fiber, few saturated fats, this slow and continuous sum of products has given rise to the now commonly called Mediterranean diet. Carbohydrates of fast and slow absorption with ample vitamins and unsaturated fats and complemented with minerals and trace elements.

The Mediterranean was the melting pot of cultures and cuisines, where everything was added. Nothing has stood out and the sun and sea have provided the strong diversity and variety It is a healthy, balanced and highly valued cuisine or diet.

Hopkin (English) together with Fujian, the 1931 Nobel Prize, found out what the essential components of a complete diet should be, and that there are other components such as vitamins that are part of the diet.

In the early twentieth century, advances in nutrition went faster than other sciences, seeking the welfare of the population.

Scientifically today the so-called Mediterranean diet is considered to be an excellent model of the role.

The Science behind the Mediterranean Diet

The cardiac disease had become a serious health problem at the turn of the 20th century. At that time, researchers studying the disease and its causes discovered a startling pattern: the incidence of heart problems was much lower in some Mediterranean countries, particularly Italy and Greece compared to America.

The basis of the Mediterranean diet

The explanation they postulated might be in their diet: rich in plants, including fruits, vegetables, whole grains, legumes, potatoes, nuts and seeds. A strong quantity of extra virgin olive oil and a modest quantity of fish, poultry, dairy and eggs, as well as red meat, rarely completed this tradition's foundation.

The scientific and nutritional interest in it is relatively recent and, like so many other items on this subject, it's supposed advantages have become almost magical forces due to the inflated word of mouth and tricky publicity.

How does the Mediterranean diet work?

A fiber-rich mixed diet with healthy fats and numerous fresh ingredients such as vegetables, Mediterranean salads, fish and fresh fruit should make our body slim. The Mediterranean diet scores with many important ingredients controlling blood lipids and reducing the risk of heart disease. Quite healthy for digestion are vegetables, fruits and salads. The menu also includes pasta, pizza, rice, legumes, cold-pressed olive oil, fresh herbs, and garlic.

The Mediterranean diet program is important: take the time to eat. So it is very important to have a slow and comfortable meal. It takes a lot of time for the Southern Europeans to cook and eat with great pleasure. Smart tactic-now studies have shown this as well: slow eating helps you lose weight. Because if you don't take your time, you also skip the natural feeling of satiety on your body and thus eat more calories unnecessarily.

Mediterranean diet also maintains healthy fat metabolism and reduces the cholesterol levels according to studies. Additionally, scientific research shows a positive correlation between the Mediterranean diet and the prevention of Alzheimer's. A US study has shown that foods such as vegetables, fruit, olive oil and the like can lower the risk of Alzheimer's disease.

The Mediterranean diet does not provide for a supplementary sports program. Calorie counting is not the order of the day, either-you can get enough of the right food. It should always be prepared freshly in the best case.

CHAPTER TWO
Living longer with a Mediterranean diet

The Mediterranean diet, supplemented with virgin olive oil or nuts such as nuts, hazelnuts and almonds, is more effective in preventing cardiovascular diseases than low-fat diets of all kinds.

We live in a society that is obsessed with seeking the elixir of eternal youth, but there is an inexorable biological reality: we are oxidizing and that is why our bodies are aging. It is up to us to faster or slower than this oxidation. There are no miracles. It is possible to live longer and in better health conditions, as long as we are willing to change certain habits.

People who adhere to a healthy diet like the traditional Mediterranean would be more likely to prevent depression, so nutrition could help treat that mental disorder, suggests an international team of researchers.

Public health, psychiatry, and nutrition specialists evaluated the role of dietary interventions in depression with the intention of developing recommendations for future psychiatric health care, as the disorder carries high social costs.

The researchers conducted a systematic review of indices and results from 41 longitudinal and cross-sectional studies on healthy diet compliance with depressive symptoms or clinical depression, which attempted to synthesize the link between food quality and disorder.

The researchers from the United Kingdom, France, Australia and Spain conclude that a diet based on fruits, vegetables, grains, fish, nuts and olive oil, but without too much meat or dairy, seems to have advantages in terms of mood.

Dr. Camille Lasalle of University College London points out the evidence that the food we eat can make a difference in reducing our risk of depression.

Experts in metabolic medicine say more rigorous and specific trials are needed to confirm evidence of the possible connection and determine whether depression can be treated with diet.

In fact it is complicated to explain the link between mood and food, as there are many factors that may be involved.

Depression can cause loss of appetite and someone who feels bad cannot take care of it as well, while happy people can be more likely to lead healthier lifestyles, including not drinking alcohol is a depressing mood known to them.

Eating bad foods, lots of sugar and highly processed foods may increase the risk of depression, which means eliminating them from the diet is important.

Research on the traditional Mediterranean diet has shown that it can reduce our risk of developing diseases like type

2 diabetes, hypertension and high cholesterol, all of which are risk factors for cardiac diseases.

The researchers have discovered that people closely following a Mediterranean diet would live longer and have less chance of gaining weight.

Health Benefits of the Mediterranean Diet

1. Lower risk of heart disease
Olive oil is the main ingredient in cooking and Mediterranean flavor. Olive oil contains monounsaturated fats, which for a healthy heart are a good component. In comparison, eating foods high in saturated fat leads to heart disease growth. Instead of butter, many Mediterranean dishes are cooked with oil and sauces and dressings include olive oil as one of the principal ingredients.

Mix various types of balsamic spoonfuls of vinegar with oil- of whatever flavor you like and you'll get a healthy salad dressing. There's no need to buy premixed dressings filled with unnecessary fats when you can create a healthy one with just a few ingredients, simply and easily. Therefore, the fresher it is, the better and a delicious salad dressing is produced if you use a little olive oil and balsamic vinegar.

2. Lower risk of having diabetes

Olive oil has many benefits for the skin. Since Mediterranean diets use it in different ways, if you follow the diet to the letter, you'll surely benefit from it. Some research studies have shown that olive oil and the Mediterranean diet, in particular, could help reduce the risk of developing type 2 diabetes.

Researchers believe a large number of rich minerals and phytochemicals in the Mediterranean diet can decrease insulin resistance and inflammation. Your body needs to successfully break down the sugars. If the body can't do this properly, the risk of suffering from type 2 diabetes could be greater.

3. Prevents hypertension

All you consume directly affects your blood pressure and there are foods in the Mediterranean diet that can help lower the pressure. Additionally, this diet consists of healthy foods that don't increase blood pressure. Genetics can play an important role in whether or not you have hypertension although it is not very good to have an unhealthy diet that contains a lot of fat and salt.

Unnecessary sodium will not be consumed in the Mediterranean diet by not eating processed foods which will increase blood pressure and hold it at very high levels. Hypertension can cause hypertension and other cardiovascular diseases so this diet can help you to reduce the serious health risks involved.

4. Prevents fatty liver disease

A diet rich in processed foods that contain salt, sugar, calories and unhealthy fats is practiced by many people. Adopting such an unhealthy diet increases the risk of developing obesity, which is the main cause of fatty liver disease. The amount of olive oil in the Mediterranean diet helps to remove many saturated fats from the diet and, at the same time, prevents fatty liver diseases.

Interestingly, the diet does not include red meat, as it contains a lot of saturated fat. Alternatively, mineral-rich chicken and fish are the meats preferred by this diet. Everything you eat and how much you eat of something the liver has difficulty processing (such as red meat) can lead to other liver diseases.

5. A potentially longer lifespan

Some studies link longevity with the Mediterranean diet. Diet can also reduce the risk of cardiovascular disease, which ultimately helps people live longer lives. Then start eating more fresh produce, nuts, seeds and olive oil to reap health benefits, including the possibility of living longer and reducing the chances of heart problems. While it is obviously desirable to start and maintain this diet in youth throughout life, research has shown that it can also have a positive effect on those who start eating it in later life.

6. Improvement of cognitive function

The research suggests a correlation between the foods present in the Mediterranean-style diet and the improvement of brain functions, as well as a lower rate of decline in mental health. As we age, cognitive functions decrease and this sometimes leads to extremely serious conditions such as Alzheimer's disease or the appearance of dementia.

It's also common to experience a mild memory loss and misunderstanding spells when you're older and this isn't considered a sign of a neurological disorder. The Mediterranean diet can help you to stay mentally active given your age, to fully enjoy life and potentially reduce the normal effects of aging.

7. Lower risk of cancer

It has also been linked to reducing the risk of developing and dying from certain types of cancer, in addition to all other serious diseases that the Mediterranean diet may help to reduce. Eating lots of fruits and vegetables is an important component of the diet, which is one of the reasons you can reduce your cancer risk-most fruits and vegetables are rich in antioxidants.

It is understood that antioxidants are anti-carcinogenic. Nuts and oils in the Mediterranean diet also play an important role in reducing inflammation and insulin differentiation, which may inhibit the growth of certain types of cancer.

8. Reduction of preservatives and chemicals

The Mediterranean diet is filled with fresh produce, vegetables and fruits, meats delivered straight from the butcher shop, and ocean-fresh fish. It means we do not consume precooked and processed foods that typically contain a lot of additives and preservatives that are not safe for anyone.

If you want to see something as simple as a frozen chicken package, there are usually multiple lines in the ingredient list you don't eat only chicken. In addition to salt, fat, sugar and calories, precooked foods bring other potentially harmful ingredients into your body. Any foods that can be harmful to your health will be eliminated following a Mediterranean-style diet.

9. Increased consumption of antioxidants

Antioxidants, nowadays, are a phenomenon. List after list of super-foods includes antioxidant-rich components.

These have been linked to lowering the risk of certain types of cancer and the benefits don't stop there-they have natural anti-inflammatory properties and can help prevent heart disease, decrease the risk of developing diabetes and boost the immune system. They also possess anti-aging properties.

That's a fantastic list of potential benefits and eating more fresh fruits and vegetables is all you need to do. Explore the various types and stuff you've never eaten before. There's no reason I couldn't explore new food!

10. Less likely to suffer from Parkinson's disease

There is some debate as to whether or not the diet in the Mediterranean style may minimize the risk of Parkinson's disease developing, but there are enough scientists who believe that there is a link worth considering.

A study published in the American Journal of Clinical Nutrition found that the development of diseases such as Parkinson's and Alzheimer's had decreased by 13 percent when participants followed a Mediterranean diet, which is a fairly large number in general terms. The exact diet portion that reduces this risk has not been established but the facts are insight.

Losing Weight with the Mediterranean Diet

There are many different types of diets, perhaps even too many. However, experts say you should pay attention to the healthiest ones, which also provide nutrients to your body in addition to helping you lose weight. Mediterranean diet-making friends with it are worthwhile, because it is a great example of this. Don't forget this approach!

The Mediterranean diet is rich in protein, fiber, omega-3 fatty acids, whole grains, minerals, vitamins, and most importantly, it contains almost no fat, carbohydrate, and industrial flour. Let's look at it deeper.

How can a Mediterranean diet help me lose weight?

- First of all, the strict Mediterranean diet is not the same as weight loss. This diet is synonymous with the development of very healthy eating habits and thanks to the ingredients found therein, we learn to control body weight and exclude everything else that can lead to weight gain and even diseases from the diet. Nutritionists suggest you can lose weight just one kilogram a week by using this type of diet.
- In other words, the Mediterranean diet is not only helpful to us but also to our entire family. The World Health Organization (WHO) proposed the basic principles of the so-called healthy eating pyramids.

- The advantages of a Mediterranean diet are the product of the excellent quantity of healthy fats. These are just monounsaturated fats that are present in olive oil and fatty acids like Omega 3 and 6.
- That diet excludes both animal protein and red meat.
- The richest in antioxidants is the Mediterranean diet: fruits, dried fruits, vegetables and legumes.
- This contains a good amount of fiber.
- The Mediterranean diet helps to reduce cholesterol in the body, protects against cardiovascular disease and takes care of your weight due to a healthy amount of nutrients that removes unhealthy fat.

CHAPTER THREE
Starting the Mediterranean Diet

The first step in getting the Mediterranean diet started is to learn its foundations, that is, the ingredients that make it up and make it one of the world's healthiest choices.

1. Olive oil as a fat preference

Rich in vitamin E, monounsaturated fatty acids and antioxidants, the Mediterranean diet's essential oil is this.

For example, it is used to season salads, fry, toast and all that needs some form of fat for seasoning or cooking!

So if you're thinking about starting the Mediterranean diet, leave the butter and heat the olive oil.

2. Daily consumption of plant foods

For their significant contribution of minerals, vitamins, fibers and antioxidants, grains, fruits, vegetables and nuts are eaten every day and regularly. However, according to the Mediterranean diet food pyramid, each main meal should include: 1-2 fruits More than 2 vegetable servings, natural or cooked. Preferably, at least one raw daily portion.

3. Daily cereal consumption

One or two portions of cereal are recommended per meal, preferably whole grain in the form of rice, pasta, bread, couscous or other types, for example. The carbohydrates derived from these foods will, of course, provide the necessary energy to face the day.

4. Choose fresh, seasonal foods

The purchasing and use of fresh and seasonal foods allow us to enjoy their nutrients, taste and fragrance. Use foods that are unprocessed and seasonal. It is a safe step and is environmentally friendly.

5. Moderate consumption of red meat

Because of the health problems that animal fat intake can create, moderate consumption of red and processed meat is recommended. Therefore, according to the Mediterranean diet, the saturated fats of these meats must be reduced.

6. Daily consumption of dairy products

Yogurt and cheese are a daily part of the Mediterranean diet and contain important minerals such as calcium and phosphorus, vitamins and proteins with a high biological value.

7. Fish two times a week and eggs, three or four

Starting with the Mediterranean diet, it's important to reduce your consumption of red meat and instead eat fish, for example, for its content of Omega-3 fatty acids and eggs, sources of quality protein.

8. Bakery and sweets products, very low consumption

It's not a matter of removing these ingredients from your diet entirely, but note that your consumption should be extremely moderate. In fact, it recommends fewer than two servings a week.

9. Water as a preferred drink

Water is a key Mediterranean diet pillar and should be your favorite drink. Furthermore, wine is also part of this diet, consumed in moderation and usual fashion.

10. Physical exercise

A good diet is not the only thing that you need to look for to enjoy good health. Therefore, n will make sure to exercise daily and regularly to enjoy the benefits of a healthy diet.

CHAPTER FOUR

Eat Well and Stay Healthy the Mediterranean Way

The Mediterranean diet is an eating style that can help you lose weight and improve your health. Typically eaten in countries and regions bordering the Mediterranean sea, it is based on diet. This emphasizes fruits, vegetables, whole grains, and legumes while including smaller amounts of meat, poultry, dairy and sweets. Several studies have shown that the Mediterranean diet will help you lose weight and reduce the risk of heart disease, cancer, Parkinson's disease, and Alzheimer's. Adopting a lifestyle and diet in a Mediterranean style will help you eat better and stay healthy.

Adopting a Mediterranean Style Diet

Use the foods more focused on plants. Eating more plant-based foods is one of the main components of the Mediterranean diet. These types of foods will make up the majority of your diet.

Foods based on plants include a wide variety of foods—some high in protein, fiber, and many vitamins and minerals.

Most of all eat: fruits, vegetables, whole grains, nuts, peas, beans, lentils... At each meal and snack you should include one or more of those food groups.

In the Mediterranean diet nuts and seeds are especially common. These contain a large amount of protein, minerals, and heart-healthy fats. Include 1–2 table cubits per serving (14.8–29.6 ml).

Citrus fruits are another prevalent plant-based food in the Mediterranean diet. Lemons, limes, oranges, and grapefruits have large amounts of vitamin C, a potent antioxidant that has been shown.

Replace butter with heart-sanctioning oils. Another trademark of the Mediterranean diet is the use of a great deal of olive oil. It is used for cooking as well as dressing up various foods.

Butter is a less nutritious choice than olive oil, since it is very high in saturated fat. Some studies have linked higher saturated fat levels to heart disease.

On the other side, olive oil is thought to be a superior and more nutritious type of fat. It is very rich in monounsaturated fats that have been linked with reduced heart disease risk.

While olive oil is a healthier fat option, it is still fat, and should be weighed when you use it. One serving is one tablespoon and the portions should be limited to two or three per day.

Red meat limit. Red meat consumption in the US is higher than in a lot of other countries. The Mediterranean diet generally only occasionally includes red meat — perhaps once or twice a month.

Red meat was associated with a range of adverse health effects when eaten in large quantities (such as heart disease and diabetes). A study recently found that high amounts of red meat are associated with a shortened life span.

Substituting other sources of protein (such as tofu, rice, nuts, or eggs) was associated with a reduced risk of heart disease and diabetes.

Include products made with low-fat dairy. The dairy products are another great source of protein found in the Mediterranean diet. During the day throw in a serving or two of them.

Low-fat dairy contains a lot of protein but there are also high amounts of calcium, vitamin D and potassium in these foods.

Yogurt, cheeses, milk or cottage cheese may be included in dairy products.

Measure the proper serving of dairy foods. Attach 1/2 cup yogurt, 1 oz cheese, or 6 oz low-fat milk to taste.

At least eat fish twice a week. The Mediterranean diet also stresses the consumption of fish and shellfish, in addition to eating several different sources of plant-based proteins.

Most diets in the Mediterranean style recommend eating at least twice a week fish or shellfish. Include dinner with a 3-4 oz serving of fish or shellfish.

Many shellfish and fish are larger in omega-3 fats. A particular type of fat was associated with a reduced risk of heart disease, a reduction in blood pressure, cholesterol and triglyceride.

All seafood is a great choice and particularly high in heart-healthy fats are fish such as salmon, tuna, mackerel, and sardines.

Cook instead of salt, with herbs and spices. Salt improves your food's taste, but using more herbs and spices like the Mediterranean diet also adds a lot of flavor to your food without the salt added. Salt increases the risk of hypertension which can lead to heart disease or stroke. Herbs have no adverse effects, and are useful in the diet.

Basil: This herb is very rich in essential oils and phenolic compounds that have anti-inflammatory properties and can relieve chronic inflammation such as arthritis. It is also rich in beta-carotene, lutein and vitamin A, which protect the body in an exceptional way against free radicals.

Marjoram: This plant was used for a wide range of ailments including colds, symptoms of menopause relief, cramps of the stomach and gas.

Oregano: This herb was associated with reducing disorders of the respiratory tract, GI disorders, PMS symptoms, and urinary tract infections. It is also high in fatty acids such as magnesium, dietary fiber, calcium, manganese, vitamin c, A and omega-3.

Peregrine: This common herb was thought to help prevent cancer, diabetes and improve the health of bones. It also contains high quantities of vitamins A, K, and C.

Sage: In addition to potentially lowering blood glucose and cholesterol levels, this herb may reduce cognitive ailments like Alzheimer's and dementia.

Thyme: This herb may be effective against infection by fungi, especially those around your toenails. It may also help to reduce acne, high blood pressure and certain cancers.

Mint: This plant can help with digestion, alleviate seasonal allergies and prevent

Rosemary: The herb will improve the immune system and aid with digestion. It has anti-inflammatory properties that can decrease the severity of asthma attacks and increase blood flow to your brain, which can enhance cognitive problems.

Garlic: This spice has been involved in numerous health benefits such as the lower risk of heart disease and artery hardening, reducing high cholesterol, lowering the risk of heart attack and lowering the risk of high blood pressure.

Indulge in a glass of wine. In addition to raising your HDL (the "healthy" cholesterol), and preserving your coronary arteries, drinking wine in moderation will reduce your chances of developing cardiovascular diseases.

Several research studies have shown that the right amounts of wine consumption— one glass (5 oz) or less per day— have its benefits.

Wine helps dilate the arteries and increase blood flow within your body. Wine phenols also aid in reducing bad cholesterol. When you drink alcohol, try drinking one 5-ounce glass of wine per day.

Eat smaller portions. The portions that are usually served in the US are much greater than required. Large large portions, when consumed, can lead to excess calorie intake, weight gain and obesity.

Smaller portions of the Mediterranean diet include. Such smaller portions can help keep calories low and reduce weight or maintain weight.

Measure portions of all groceries. To stay on track, you can use a food scale, or weigh cups. Guessing or "eye-balling" portions usually results in larger portions than is required.

Protein foods should be 3-4 oz per serving, vegetables 1 cup or 2 cups of leafy greens, fruit 1/2 cup and grains 1/2 cup per serving as well.

Exercise regularly. People are far more involved in the countries bordering the Mediterranean than in the US. Their increased level of activity is partly the reason why they consider their lifestyle very healthy.

Physical activity has been associated with many health benefits, including increased levels of high-density lipoprotein (HDL or "healthy" cholesterol), decreased levels of triglycerides, decreased risk of diabetes and high blood pressure, enhanced arthritis-related pain, and decreased cancer rates.

Seek to do aerobic exercise of moderate intensity at least for 30 minutes during each session five days a week. This will help you meet the US minimum physical activity requirement of 150 minutes per week.

Take up walking, running, cycling, swimming, and hiking to get aerobic exercise. Include two to three days of 20-minute strength training every week.

You should also try pilates or yoga that will help build your strength and flexibility.

Walk and move more throughout the day. People living in the Mediterranean are taking part in more leisure practices compared to people living in the US. It has been shown that being more active over the day has similar benefits to aerobic activity.

Lifestyle practice is the activity that you embed in your daily routine. Taking the stairs, for example, or mopping down the concrete, are called lifestyle behaviors.

Throughout their days' Mediterranean people tend to have more activity in the lifestyle. For instance, we're cycling to and from destinations, or riding a bike instead. Involvement is an essential part of your daily routine.

Think of your day, the schedule for your work and the whole week. Where can you put in more movement or more steps? Can you ride a motorcycle to work? Can you go to the drugstore or grocery store? You should take the stairs instead of the lift? Try to incorporate more moves into your day.

Eat mindfully. Another feature of a Mediterranean diet and lifestyle is that they usually eat more carefully compared to the American hustle and bustle. Conscious eating can help eat less, enjoy eating more and even help you lose weight.

It's a way to eat carefully. It's a way to eat that makes you more aware of what kind of food you consume, how much you eat and how easily you eat.

Take 20 minutes to eat your meal, remove distractions from your dining area (e.g., TVs or cell phones), take small bites, chew more thoroughly, and adjust your body's sense of satiety.

Manage stress. Chronic lifestyle stress can be tough to deal with. Studies have shown, however, that people living in Mediterranean countries can deal with stress better and suffer less from heart disease.

Try to tackle as much tension as possible. Try to listen to music, exercise, meditate, do yoga, or converse with a friend or family member.

When stress management is too complicated, or if you are unsure how to deal with stress, see a life coach or therapist for additional assistance.

When talking about the Mediterranean diet, the evolution of the human species over the centuries must be taken into account, which has brought about many changes both in their way of life and in their relationship with the rest of the species, as well as in the transformation of their diet reflected in changes in food depending on geographical areas.

In human history there has been a long transition from prehistoric hunters and gatherers to the present day. Throughout post-industrialized societies, major changes have occurred which are also reflected in the diet and nature of human nutrition.

In different cultures it is possible to recognize certain features that make their diet a lifestyle. This is done with the popular Mediterranean diet, a diet that combines various ingredients from local agriculture through recipes and special methods of healthy cooking.

Instead of a food program, the popular and world-famous Mediterranean diet is a cultural heritage that encourages you to lead a healthy lifestyle consisting of a variety of ingredients used to prepare recipes focused on exercise in seasonal, natural, and local items with moderate physical activity.

As its name suggests, this diet is born in the villages of the Mediterranean basin, transmitted from generation to generation for centuries and changing and incorporating new techniques of food and cultivation according to the geographical location of these populations.

The Mediterranean Diet's basic ingredients make up a perfect "wheat-vine-olive" triangle to which vegetables, legumes, fruits, fish, cheeses, and nuts are added and olive oil is the main source of fats. The Mediterranean Diet offers enough macronutrients to the body through a healthy and varied diet plan.

CHAPTER FIVE
Mediterranean Diet Food Pyramid Vs Traditional Food Pyramid

For most of us, the food pyramid contains the most recognized symbol of healthy food. This demonstrates which foods we can consume in which portion size so our body gets the nutrients these needs. If you are designing a healthy diet plan you will do well to look at the pyramid of Mediterranean diet foods.

What is the Mediterranean Diet Food Pyramid?

The Mediterranean diet food pyramid is an alternative to the conventional one that is becoming increasingly popular because it is not based on popular trends in the food industry. The diet itself is centered within the Mediterranean region, on thousands of years of tradition. Mediterranean countries ' dietary traditions have long been recognized as being very healthy, and the food they eat is one of the main factors in that healthiness. Being aware of the difference between the traditional food pyramid and the Mediterranean one will help you improve your health.

The Mediterranean diet pyramid is substantially different from the traditional one we are familiar with. Several glaring discrepancies, namely;

- The Mediterranean one has no fats category Red meat is at the top of the Mediterranean pyramid as a food to eat with sweets / desserts at least.
- Olive oil is grouped with fruit and vegetables as something to be frequently consumed

The top portion of the Mediterranean diet food pyramid starts with red meat as an animal protein source. Red meat and candy are the Mediterranean's least-eaten foods, around 2-3 times a month. The next group, eaten a few days a week, includes meat, eggs and dairy products such as cheese and yogurt. Next come fish and seafood eaten almost daily. The Mediterranean diet is basically low in saturated fats and high in monounsaturated fats, and high in omega 3.

The lower pyramid level consists of fruits, vegetables, legumes (beans), nuts, seeds, herbs, spices, whole-grain bread, whole-grain pasta, couscous, brown rice, polenta, and other whole grains. The Mediterranean people rarely eat processed grains (i.e., white flour). A wide number of these fresh foods are consumed every day, and are usually either raw or cooked slightly. Which ensures nutrients remain intact. Cooking foods actually kills or makes most nutrients indigestible. Hence eating raw or partially cooked food is always safer.

The main aspect of the Mediterranean pyramid is to prescribe six glasses of water per day and a moderate amount of wine (i.e. one glass of red wine with dinner).

It is interesting to note that in the Mediterranean pyramid, olive oil is grouped with fruits and vegetables. As you can imagine, olive oil is an essential part of the Mediterranean diet and includes many dishes. While it is true that oil is high in calories, olive oil is a good, monounsaturated fat that is high in antioxidants and contains omega-3 fatty acids, so we can consume a little more as long as we don't go crazy. Monounsaturated oils like olive oil are anti-inflammatory and help with diseases like asthma and arthritis. These are also safer in the heart because Omega 3 lowers LDL ("bad") cholesterol and increases HDL ("good") cholesterol. Less natural olive oil.

You may wonder how Mediterranean people receive their iron, as they don't eat a lot of red meat. The response to this is the same as a vegetarian is. Also good sources of iron are legumes (beans) and green leafy vegetables, and the Mediterranean diet is full of these healthy foods. Nevertheless, the whole Mediterranean diet food pyramid is made up of healthy foods that ensure that those who adopt the Mediterranean diet enjoy optimal health.

How to Implement the Mediterranean Diet into Your Lifestyle

We are all involved in being lean, losing weight, getting a good diet plan, getting rid of cardiovascular and health-related illnesses. Typically, once you have a good diet plan such as the Mediterranean diet pan, the chances are that you will eventually reduce the number of calories in your body resulting in decreased heart-related issues.

The other benefits include weight shedding, fat burning and gradually slimming down. It is truly easy to implement diet plans like the Mediterranean diet plan. That's because you can't eat the gunk and bland vegetables that many people have to submit to just because they want to live longer and healthier.

You will enjoy delicious meals with the Mediterranean diet plan while still rising the chances of getting heart-related problems. Here are a few tips to help adopt the Mediterranean diet.

1. Decide on What Diet Type

Most of the people tend to worry about their diet plans consistently. They worry if it will work if they lose weight if they can reduce their chances of dying younger as a result of heart disease and cancer and, most importantly, worry if they can keep up with their diets. Okay, the thing is, if you really want to do this, you have to choose which choice you think works best for you.

There are two main dietary forms or regimens. You can do the form planned or the style Do-It-Yourself. It all depends on the makeup you have. For instance, some people don't like strict time tables and are more likely to fail to use them because they are instinctively opposed to things that make them feel like they're boxed in.

Though, other people find it exciting to chart a strategy and are more likely to stick to it. It all depends on the person that you are. So, whatever happens, just pick one out. If you don't know which group you're moving for, just go for one. You can always turn to the other, if you don't like it.

2. Find Recipes that Will Work for You

The taste of the people in the food is different. You need to find and stick to that which works for you. The basic components of the Mediterranean diet plan include, among others, olive oil, legumes, vegetables, nuts, grains, unprocessed carbohydrates, fish, reduced red meat consumption and saturated fat.

Now, if you just like eating them like that, then it's all right. But if you want to make it much more fun, you'd have to find recipes that work. The South Beach Diet recipes, for example, are great and fun to cook. So, find recipes that inculcate these and which are based on the Mediterranean diet.

3. Get Creative With the Diet

Since following a few diet plans, the reason many people return to eating junk is that the diets are either dull, repetitive or lacking in flavor. So, what you should do is just go for those delicious meals. Get yourself creative with the recipes. Try something new, and something different. Chances are if you're looking well enough, you'll find lots of Mediterranean diet recipes that will last you for a whole year and more.

4. Be Disciplined

Because the Mediterranean diet is really simple to use and apply, it is hardly called a diet by some. I just see it as an alternative lifestyle and food choices that help you stay healthy and live longer. The secret, then, is discipline. Stay focused and who knows, you could just give yourself an extra 15 years of health and life.

CHAPTER SIX
Reasons Why a Mediterranean Diet in the 21st Century Is A Healthy Choice

If you're a person on a quest for a solid diet plan, you may feel exhausted a lot of the time. It is almost impossible for a person to turn on a TV set or open a newspaper in the 21st century, without being bombarded with ads for a variety of different diet plans and items.

With the vast number of diet plans, services, supplements and aids on the market, a diet plan that can and will better meet your needs now and into the future may seem almost impossible to choose. Most significantly, it can be difficult to discern whether one or the other of these different diet plans are actually a healthy path to follow. In many cases, fad diets are not really focused on the foundations of a healthy life.

When you decide what sort of diet plan or a diet plan or diet will best serve your needs and enhance your health in the future, you will want to look at the benefits that the Mediterranean diet can offer.

While there are multiple reasons why a balanced alternative is a Mediterranean diet, there are five main reasons why a good choice is a Mediterranean diet.

1. The benefits of fruits, vegetables, fiber and whole grains

Regular consumption of fresh fruit and vegetables is an important component of the Mediterranean diet. Medical experts and nutritionists generally agree that a person should eat around 5-6 servings of fresh fruit and vegetables (or steamed items) daily.

People who generally adhere to the Mediterranean diet eventually eat more than the minimum recommended amount of fruit and vegetables. As a result, nutritionists in different parts of the world have prescribed a Mediterranean-based program for its customers. Today doctors who recommend healthy eating habits to their patients often stick to the Mediterranean diet.

The Mediterranean diet contains healthy amounts of dietary fiber and whole grains, in addition to fruit and vegetables. Fiber and whole grains have proven effective in reducing heart disease incidence and certain types of cancer.

2. The benefits of olive oil - avoiding saturated fat

Many people have a simple misperception of the Mediterranean diet. The Mediterranean diet is high in fat, many people have heard. There is some reality in the definition, on some point, that the Mediterranean diet is higher in fat than some other diet programs. A person who follows the Mediterranean diet takes from fat about thirty percent of their daily calories. (Most diets advised the consumption of fat calories at a rate of approximately thirteen to fifteen percent per day. Moreover, some diets envisage the intake of animal fat.)

The vast majority of the fat a person consumes on the Mediterranean diet comes from olive oil. The fat present in the Mediterranean diet is not, in other words, the unhealthy saturated fat that can cause disease, obesity and other health concerns. Nonetheless, research has shown that there are a variety of solid benefits of olive oil consumption, including a decrease in the risk of breast cancer incidence in women.

3. Dairy in moderation

While in some cases it can be helpful to eat low-fat or non-fat dairy products, many people worldwide rely on heavy creams, eggs, and other fatty dairy products for their daily diets. The Mediterranean diet has low milk content. All dairy products which are currently on the menu are actually low in fat. A person who consumes four eggs a week is considered an extremely heavy eater of the eggs.

4. Red Meat in Moderation

Very little red meat is included in the Mediterranean diet. This diet depends on moderate amounts of lean poultry and fresh fish when it comes to meat products. As a result, people on the Mediterranean diet have lower levels of "bad" cholesterol and higher levels of "good: cholesterol". Furthermore, thanks to the inclusion of lean and fresh fish in the diet, the members of the Mediterranean diet enjoy the antioxidant benefits present in some oils and fish products.

5. A Well Balanced Dieting Scheme

Ultimately, the Mediterranean diet is gaining worldwide acclaim from experts and adherents as it is a balanced diet program. Study after study shows that a balanced diet low in fat which includes fruit, vegetables, whole grains and lean meatworks to ensure complete health and well-being.

A weekly menu based on the Mediterranean diet

Monday

- Breakfast: Coffee with milk. Toast with goat cheese spread. Apple.
- Mid-morning: cereal bar. Natural Orange Juice
- Food: Chickpea soup. Hake meatballs stewed with potatoes. Grapes.
- Snack: Cottage cheese with sugar.
- Dinner: Swiss chard with garlic. Grilled turkey and tomato cherry skewers with couscous. Custard apple.

Tuesday

- Breakfast: Milk with cocoa powder. Whole grains
- Mid-morning: Natural pear smoothie.
- Food: Stewed green beans. Grilled chicken fillet with steamed broccoli. Pineapple Carpaccio.
- Snack: Toast with quince jam.
- Dinner: Salad with cucumber, black olives, onion, and Feta cheese. Salmon with papillote vegetables. Peach.

Wednesday

- Breakfast: Milk Crispbread with strawberry jam.
- Mid-morning: Sandwich with lettuce, tomato, and cheese. Natural grape juice.

- Food: Tomato soup. Broth rice with rabbit and artichokes. Orange.
- Snack: Seed bread with olive oil.
- Dinner: Cauliflower sauteed with bacon. Scrambled eggs with roasted mushrooms. Banana with yogurt.

Thursday

- Breakfast: Milk Olive bread with slices of tomato and virgin olive oil.
- Mid-morning: Apple compote.
- Food: Roasted red peppers with pine nuts. Grilled pork loin with mustard and rice sauce. Khaki.
- Snack: Tuna mini sandwich.
- Dinner: Vegetable cream with croutons. Fried fish. Tangerines

Friday

- Breakfast: Coffee with milk. Toast with chocolate spread.
- Mid-morning: Muesli with dried fruit.
- Food: Stewed beans. Tortilla with vegetables and peas (Campesina) with lettuce. Grapes.
- Snack: Milk. Homemade cake.

- Dinner: Sauteed Brussels sprouts with chopped almonds. Spinach, goat cheese and honey crepe with zucchini slices. Pear.

Saturday

- Breakfast: Integral cookies. Pineapple yogurt smoothie.
- Mid-morning: Appetizer: assorted montaditos.
- Food: Migas. Nice pickled with onion. Banana flambé with chocolate.
- Snack: Macedonia.
- Dinner: Two-color puree (potato and beet) gratin. Baked carrot chicken thighs. Orange.

Sunday

- Breakfast: Coffee with milk. Ensaimada
- Mid-morning: Appetizer: assorted nuts, dried fruits, and olives.
- Food: Vegetable cannelloni au gratin. Grilled duck breast with fig sauce. Orange with custard
- Snack: Apple rolled with cinnamon.
- Dinner: Fine noodle soup. Eggs stuffed with smoked salmon gratin with grated carrot. Fruit frozen yogurt.

CHAPTER SEVEN
Mediterranean breakfast recipes

- Scrambled eggs with truffles

Ingredients

- 100 g shrimp (peeled and cooked)
- 3 egg yolks
- 125 ml of milk
- 125 ml whipped cream
- Sea salt (from the mill)
- Pepper (white, from the mill)
- 1 tbsp truffle oil

Preparation

1. Whisk the milk, cream, egg yolk and truffle oil in a stainless steel bowl, stirring constantly with hot steam until the egg begins to freeze.
2. Roughly chop the prawns and stir into the truffle.
3. Season the truffle eggshell with freshly ground salt and pepper.

- Spaghettiomelett

Ingredients

- 5 eggs
- 150 g spaghetti
- 30 g parmesan (freshly grated)
- 30 g butter
- 1 pinch of nutmeg (grated)
- Sea salt
- Pepper

Preparation

1. Cook and strain the spaghetti according to the package as required.
2. Beat the eggs in a bowl. Stir in the parmesan and season with salt, pepper and a pinch of nutmeg.
3. Mix in cooked spaghetti and stir well.
4. Fry half of the butter in a pan and fry the pasta mixture in a golden heat without stirring.
5. Melt the remaining butter on top of the omelet. Turn the omelet over and fry the other side until crispy.
6. Portion and serve hot.

- Croque Monsieur

Ingredients

- 2 eggs
- 1 pinch paprika powder

- 1 pinch of chili pepper (or grated nutmeg)
- Oil (for baking)
- 8 slices of toasted bread
- 4 slices of Gryère cheese (alternatively Emmental cheese)
- 4 slices of ham (or 8 slices of bacon)
- 200 ml of milk

Preparation

1. For the Croque Monsieur, the top half of the toast with a slice of cheese and ham or 2 slices of bacon. Cover each with a slice of bread. Mix the eggs with milk, paprika powder, chili or nutmeg on a deep plate.
2. Pour oil into a pan about finger-high and heat. Briefly turn the filled toasts in the egg-milk on both sides and bake in the hot oil on both sides with the lowest possible heat and with the lid closed until the cheese has melted and the toasts are a nice golden yellow. Lift out and dab the Croque Monsieur well before serving.

- Crab choux

Ingredients

- 250 g crabs (small, in the shell)
- 250 g flour

- 1 tbsp butter
- 4 eggs
- salt
- Vegetable oil (for baking)
- Parsley (for sprinkling)

Preparation

1. Bring the crabs in a bit of saltwater to a boil, lift them out, let them cool down and peel. Squeeze about 200 ml of cooking water through a hair strainer and bring in a saucepan to boil. Remove the butter and flour and keep simmering, stirring constantly until the dough comes off the surface. Remove the pan from the hob and continue beating the dough until it has cooled a little. Then add one egg slowly at a time and beat vigorously again. Add crabs, and let the dough rest for 15 minutes at least. Heat oil in a large saucepan. Cut the little donuts out of the dough and bake them in hot oil, golden yellow. Lift out, drain on paper in the kitchen, and sprinkle with parsley to serve.

- Greek yogurt with honeycomb

Ingredients

- 500 g yogurt (Greek)

- 150 g honeycomb
- 4 pieces of figs (fresh)
- 2 tbsp pine nuts
- Cassis syrup (black currant syrup)

Preparation

1. Peel the figs cut them into wedges and mix them with the yogurt. Roast the pine nuts, chop them and also pour them into the yogurt. Arrange yogurt in a bowl and drizzle with a little honey and cassis syrup.

- Tramezzini with egg and anchovies

Ingredients

- 12 slices of tramezzini bread (soft, juicy white bread without rind)
- 6 eggs (hard-boiled and thinly sliced)
- 12 anchovy fillets (inlaid)
- 200 g mayonnaise (homemade if possible)

Preparation

1. Brush the bread slices generously with mayonnaise. The top half of the bread with half of the egg slices. Place the drained anchovy fillets on top and top with the remaining egg slices. Put the remaining

bread slices on top and cut diagonally into two triangles.

- Herb omelet

Ingredients

- 12 eggs
- 12 tbsp herbs (of your choice, washed, finely chopped)
- 6 tablespoons of butter
- 1 tablespoon of flour
- 1/8 l milk
- salt
- pepper
- 2 tbsp parmesan (or other hard cheese to taste)

Preparation

1. For the herbal omelet, first, melt the butter in a pan and gently braise the herbs on a low flame. Attention: The herbs must not brown at all!
2. In the meantime, stir the eggs with salt, pepper, parmesan, flour, and milk into a liquid pancake batter. Pour carefully over the herbs, stir well. When a firm crust has formed on the underside, turn the dough and bake. (Add a little butter to taste, so that the other side also becomes crispy.)

3. Arrange and serve the herb omelet on plates.

Tip

1. The herbal omelet can be eaten hot, is cut into pie-like triangles but is also perfect as a small bite with wine. The herbal omelet is also ideal as a soup inlay! In this function - a little modified and cut into small strips - it has also made a career in Viennese cuisine as a "fried soup".

- **Caprese Toast**

Ingredients

- 1-2 paradises
- 2 pkg. Mozzarella
- 1 clove of garlic
- 4 slices of toast
- 1 tbsp pesto (basil)
- 1 tablespoon of olive oil
- Basil (fresh)
- salt
- Pepper (from the mill)

Preparation

1. For the Caprese toast, first, wash the parsnip and cut it into slices. Also, cut the mozzarella into slices. Peel garlic and chop finely.
2. Brush the toast slices with pesto and place the parsnip and mozzarella on top. Mix the garlic and olive oil and spread over them.
3. Bake the toasts with the grill function of the oven until the mozzarella melts.
4. Salt and pepper the Caprese toast before serving and garnish with fresh basil leaves.

- Italian rolls ("pane arabo")

Ingredients

- 500 g of flour
- 300 g water (lukewarm)
- 1 pkg. Of dry yeast
- 1 tsp salt (coated)
- 1 tsp sugar (coated)

Preparation

1. Mix the flour, yeast, salt, sugar, and water and knead well. It should be an elastic and not sticky dough. Knead in a little more flour if necessary. Leave the dough covered until it has doubled (approx. 1 hour).

2. Divide the dough into 8 parts and roll them out with a rolling pin to round or oval rolls. Place the rolls on a baking sheet lined with baking paper and cover them with a clean kitchen towel and let them rise for another 30 minutes.
3. Preheat the oven to 250 ° C.
4. Bake the rolls for about 10-12 minutes. From the 8th minute, check again and again that the rolls are not too brown.
5. The rolls can still be served warm.

- Eggs alla Saltimbocca

Ingredients

- 4 eggs
- Pepper (black, freshly ground)
- 4 slices of Parma ham
- 8 sage leaves (large)
- 2 tablespoons of olive oil
- 4 toothpicks

Preparation

1. Bring water to a boil in a saucepan and boil the eggs for 6 to 7 minutes until they are soft to the touch. Let the eggs cool, remove the shell and cut in half lengthways. Pepper the cut surfaces.
2. Halve the length of the ham and wrap a strip around half an egg.
3. Wash the sage leaves, pat dry and attach each leaf to the ham with a toothpick.
4. Heat the oil in a pan and fry the wrapped eggs over moderate heat for about 5 minutes until the ham is crispy. Turn the eggs.
5. Place two egg halves on a plate and serve immediately.

- Oatmeal Seasoned with Vegetables

Instructions

- 4 cups of water
- 2 cups of "cut" oatmeal (quick-cooking steel-cut oats)
- 1 teaspoon Italian spices
- ½ teaspoon Herbamare or sea salt
- 1 teaspoon garlic powder
- 1 teaspoon onion powder
- ½ cup nutritional yeast
- ¼ teaspoon turmeric powder

- 1½ cup kale or tender spinach
- ½ cup sliced mushrooms
- ¼ cup grated carrots
- ½ cup small chopped peppers

Preparations

1. Boil the water in a saucepan.
2. Add the oatmeal and spices and lower the temperature.
3. Cook over low heat without lid for 5 to 7 minutes.
4. Add the vegetables.
5. Cover and set aside for 2 minutes.
6. Serve immediately.

- Millo and flaxseed pancakes

These delicious pancakes are fluffy and popular with adults and children! Everyone keeps coming back for more. The combination of almond milk and rice vinegar creates the buttery taste that people crave.

Instructions

- 3 cups oatmeal
- ½ cup of millet flour
- ½ cup ground flax seeds
- 1 teaspoon of sea salt
- 1½ teaspoon baking soda
- 2 teaspoons baking powder

- 4 cups vanilla almond milk
- 2 tablespoons rice vinegar
- 1 tablespoon maple honey or date paste
- 1 tablespoon pure vanilla extract
- 3 tablespoons unsweetened applesauce

Preparations

1. Mix the dry ingredients in a bowl.
2. In a different bowl, mix the liquid ingredients.
3. Pour the liquid ingredients over the dry ones and combine them well.
4. Process the mixture well in a blender until smooth and lump-free.
5. Heat a pan over medium-low heat.
6. Using a ladle, pour the desired amount of mixture into the pan.
7. Turn the pancake when bubbles appear on the top, and underneath it is firm for approximately 5 minutes.

- Millet and buckwheat muffins with black currants

Ingredient

- ½ cup (90 g) of millet
- ½ cup (80 g) of unroasted buckwheat groats
- 4 chopped figs

- ¾ cup (160 ml) oatmeal or rice milk
- 1 tablespoon applesauce
- 1 heaped tablespoon (40 g) peanut butter
- 1 large ripe banana
- 1 pinch of sea salt
- 2 heaped teaspoons of baking powder
- ¾ cup (100 g) blackcurrants, fresh or frozen

Preparations

1. Dip millet and buckwheat overnight (or all day) in separate containers. Wash and drain (a filter can be used).
2. Soak the chopped figs in ¾ cup (160 ml) of oat milk for at least 30 minutes.
3. Heat the oven to 300-350 ° F (177 ° C).
4. Put the ingredients, except baking powder and blackcurrants, in a blender and mix them until a homogeneous lump is formed without lumps. Do not worry; It is supposed to be quite liquid since millet inflates considerably.
5. Now mix the baking powder. Unplug the blender and finally combine (DON'T LIQUID) the currants with a spoon.
6. Divide the dough into 9 muffin pans and bake for 33 to 35 minutes, until golden brown.

Apple and pumpkin pie

Ingredient

- 1 spoon ground flax seeds + 2 ½ tablespoons water (flax egg)
- ½ cup all-purpose gluten-free flour (or oatmeal)
- 1 ½ cup quick-cooking oatmeal
- 1 tablespoon baking powder
- 1 teaspoon baking soda
- 2 tablespoons pumpkin pie spice
- 1 tablespoon cinnamon
- 4 medium granny smith apples
- ½ cup date pasta
- 1 cup pumpkin puree
- 1 teaspoon vanilla extract
- ¼ cup of water (optional)

Preparations

1. Preheat the oven to 350 degrees F.
2. Mix ground flaxseed (flax) seeds with water in a small bowl and set aside for 10 minutes.
3. Mix all dry ingredients in a large bowl.
4. Cut the apples into thin slices and place them in a container.
5. Add the pumpkin puree, vanilla extract, flaxseed with water, and date paste to apples and mix well.

6. merge the dry ingredients with the apples and mix well. Add water if the mixture seems to be too dry.
7. Place the mixture in an 8 x 11 (2 quarts) container suitable for baking and bake for 30-35 minutes.

- Pumpkin and oatmeal bars

Ingredient

- 3 cups thick oatmeal
- 1 cup seedless dates
- ½ cup of boiling water
- 2 teaspoons pumpkin pie spice
- 1 tablespoon ground flaxseed or chia seeds
- ¼ cup small sliced nuts (optional)
- ¼ cup of vegetable milk
- 1 cup mashed pumpkin

Preparations

1. Preheat the oven to 350 degrees Fahrenheit.
2. Cut the date into small pieces, put them in a bowl, and pour hot water. Rest for 10 minutes.
3. Add dry ingredients to the bowl and mix well.
4. Add dates to the dry ingredients along with water, pumpkins, and plant milk and mix well.
5. Cover the square bread with baking paper and push the mixture firmly into the bread.

6. Cook for 15-20 minutes.
7. Allow the mixture to cool completely in the container, then cut into 16 squares or 8 large bars.
8. Store in the refrigerator for up to 7 days.

- Blackberry and lemon muffins for tea

Ingredient

- 2 cups whole grain wheat flour for baking
- ½ cup of Sucanat (refined cane sugar)
- 1½ teaspoon baking powder
- 1 teaspoon grated lemon peel
- ½ cup natural soy yogurt
- 1 cup non-dairy milk
- 1 tablespoon lemon juice
- 2 egg substitutes (2 tablespoons ground flaxseed with 6 tablespoons water)
- 1 cup blackberries
- 2 tablespoons coconut with reduced-fat and sugar-free content (optional)

Preparation

1. Preheat to 350 ° F (177 ° C) in the oven.
2. Fill a paper-coated mold for 12 muffins (or use a non-stick skillet).

3. In a medium bowl, mix flour, sucanat sweetener, baking powder, and rubbed lemon peel.
4. In a separate bowl, mix soy yogurt, milk, lemon juice, and egg substitutes.
5. Pour into the dry mixture the wet mixture and stir until it is hot.
6. Carefully add blackberries.
7. In the prepared muffin pan, distribute the mixture evenly.
8. Sprinkle the coconut (optional) on top of the muffins.
9. Bake them for 45 minutes in the preheated oven or until one of them has a toothpick inserted in the middle. Until serving, let them cool slightly.

- **Cocoa, banana, and whole-grain spelled flour muffins**

Ingredient

- 2 large bananas (I use frozen bananas and then defrost them)
- 2 cups whole grain spelled flour
- 1 cup walnuts, chopped into large pieces
- ½ cup raw cocoa powder
- ¼ cup applesauce
- 1 cup almond milk

- ¼ cup maple syrup, 100% pure
- ½ teaspoon baking powder

Preparations

1. Preheat the oven to 300-350 ° F (177 ° C).
2. Line the muffin pan with baking paper.
3. Crush the bananas in a large bowl.
4. Add the almond milk, maple syrup, applesauce, and mix them.
5. Add whole-grain spelled flour, baking powder, and cocoa powder and mix them.
6. Add the chopped walnuts.
7. Pour the mixture into muffin pans.
8. Cook the muffins for about 25 minutes or until when a skewer is inserted, it is clean.

Oatmeal and Apple Muffins

Ingredient

- 1 cup unsweetened applesauce
- ¼ to ½ cup of seedless dates
- 1 cup oat milk (you can use another non-dairy milk)
- Egg substitute (2 tablespoons of flaxseed mixed with 6 tablespoons of water)
- 1 tablespoon apple cider vinegar
- ½ cup unrefined sugar

- 1 teaspoon cinnamon
- 1 ½ cups oat flakes
- ½ cup raisins
- 1½ cup whole grain wheat flour
- ¾ teaspoon baking soda
- 1 teaspoon baking powder

Preparations

1. The oven should be preheated to 300-375 ° F (191 ° C).
2. Puree with 1/4 to 1/2 cup of seedless dates with 1 cup of applesauce (depending on the desired sweetness).
3. Mix the linseed with water in a large bowl. Applesauce, milk, sugar, raisins, and vinegar are added; blend well. Add the oatmeal, stir and set aside until all is combined.
4. Place the flour, baking soda, and baking powder into a separate bowl. Apply it to the mixture of apple and oatmeal and whisk until all is combined.
5. Pour the mixture into a lightly oiled silicone muffin mold with a spoon. (If you're using a regular muffin pan, cupcake papers should be used).
6. Bake the muffins till they are ready for 20 to 25 minutes.

- Pear and hazelnut crostini

Ingredients

- 4-8 slices of spelled bread (or baguette)
- 3 pears (Good Helene)
- 2 tbsp hazelnuts (chopped)
- 200 g yogurt (Greek)
- 3 tbsp maple syrup
- lemon balm

Preparation

1. First, stir in the yogurt with 2 tablespoons of maple syrup. Wash, peel, core and cut the pears into thin slices.
2. Toast bread slices or fry them in a pan with olive oil.
3. Brush the bread with yogurt, top with the pear slices and sprinkle with the hazelnuts and lemon balm.
4. Drizzle the remaining maple syrup over the pear and hazelnut crostini and serve the crostini.

- Feta and olive pancakes with bird salad

Ingredients

For the salad:

- 1 cup (s) bird salad (washed and dried)
- 3 tbsp cashew nuts (roasted)
- Apple Cider Vinegar
- olive oil
- sea-salt
- Pepper (from the mill)

For the pancakes:

- 100 g milk
- 200 g yogurt (Greek)
- 1 tbsp baking powder
- 1 tsp soda
- 150 g flour (smooth)
- 3 eggs
- 3 tbsp olives (black, chopped)
- 2 sprig (s) of thyme (leaves plucked)
- 100 g feta (crumbled)
- sea-salt
- Pepper (from the mill)
- Olive oil (for frying)

Preparation

1. Stir the milk, butter, baking powder, baking soda, flour and eggs for the pancakes first with feta olive pancakes and bird salad. Remove the olives, feta and thyme and season with salt and pepper.

2. In a saucepan heat the olive oil and fry the pancake mixture in 3 to 4 portions (thaler should not be too large). Turn and bake for 1 minute once bubbles have formed.
3. Mix the bird salad and the cashew nuts, season with a little vinegar of apple cider, olive oil, sea salt and pepper.
4. Mount the pancakes into a tower and serve with bird salad on the feta olive pancakes.

Bruschetta with mozzarella

Ingredients

- 1/4 kg tomatoes (diced)
- 2 cloves of garlic (finely chopped)
- 1 pinch of salt
- some pepper
- 1 pinch paprika powder
- 1-2 mozzarella
- 1 handful of basil (chopped)
- some olive oil
- 1 loaf (s) of ciabatta (cut into slices approximately thumb-wide)
- some sugar

Preparation

1. For the bruschetta with mozzarella, fry the tomatoes and garlic in a hot pan with olive oil.
2. Season with salt, pepper, paprika powder, sugar, and basil and let it brew for another 5 minutes.
3. Place the hot bruschetta on the ciabatta, place the finely chopped mozzarella on top and let it melt and garnish with basil.

- Greek omelet

Ingredients

- 4 eggs
- 150 g feta
- 2 tablespoons of olive oil
- Oregano (dried)
- Chives (finely chopped)
- Basil leaves (fresh)

Preparation

1. For the Greek omelet, pat the feta cheese dry with kitchen paper and cut into small cubes or crumble.

2. Pour oil into the hot pan and add whisked eggs. Then sprinkle the chopped feta cheese evenly over it.
3. Slowly slow down on a low flame, sprinkle with dried oregano. Divide the omelet in half, fold it together and sprinkle with chives on the plates.
4. Decorate with fresh basil leaves. Serve with bread and salad. Be sure to have pepper and salt grinder at the table.

- Masabacha green lentil curry

Ingredients

- 3 tablespoons of extra virgin olive oil
- 1 small onion, finely diced
- 1 ½ teaspoon of chopped garlic
- ⅔ cup of green lentils, rinsed
- ⅔ cup of red lentils, rinsed
- 2 cups of low-sodium no-chicken or chicken broth
- 1-2 cups of water, divided
- 1 ½ teaspoon of curry powder
- 1 medium-sized carrot, roughly grated
- ¼ teaspoon of kosher salt
- ¼ teaspoon of ground pepper
- 1 cup of thinly sliced arugula
- 2 tablespoons of finely chopped red onion

- 1 jalapeño pepper, sliced
- ⅔ cup of tahini
- 1 ½ teaspoon of chopped garlic
- ½ cup of ice water
- ¼ cup of lemon juice
- ¼ teaspoon of kosher salt

Preparation

1. Heat oil over medium heat, in a medium saucepan. Add the onion and cook, stirring for 5 to 8 minutes, until tender and translucent. Add the garlic and cook for 1-3 minutes, stirring. Add lentils, broth, 1 cup water, and curry powder, green and red. After high heat brings to a boil. Reduce heat to cook for 15 minutes and keep a simmer.
2. Stir in carrot and cook, stirring occasionally and add 2 tablespoons of water at a time if appropriate, until the green lentils are tender and the red lentils have broken down, 20 to 25 minutes more. Put away from heat, and add salt and pepper to taste. Cover. Cover.
3. Meanwhile, to prepare tahini sauce: in a mini food processor, combine tahini and garlic. In a slow stream add ice water with the motor running. Process, about 1 minute, until the tahini is light and fluffy. Add lemon juice and salt; process for about 30 seconds, until smooth.

4. Divide the lentil mixture on each plate between 4 plates, and dollop 2 tablespoons of tahini sauce. Arugula, red onion, and jalapeño top the lentils. Serve with the additional tahini sauce, if you wish.

- Mushroom olive frittata

Ingredients

- 1 tablespoon of olive oil
- 1 cup of sliced fresh cremini mushrooms
- 2 cups of roughly chopped fresh Swiss chard or spinach
- 1 large shallot, cut into thin slices
- 4 eggs
- 2 proteins
- 2 teaspoons of sliced fresh rosemary or 1/2 teaspoon of dried rosemary, crushed
- ¼ teaspoon of ground black pepper
- ⅛ teaspoon of salt
- ¼ cup of thinly sliced kalamata olives
- ⅓ cup of grated parmesan

Preparation

1. Cover broiler with preheating. Heat the oil over medium heat in a broiler-proof medium-nonstick skillet. Add mushrooms to skillet; cook, stirring occasionally, for 3 minutes. Add shallot and Swiss chard. Cook, stirring occasionally, about 5 minutes or until mushrooms and chard are tender.
2. Alternatively, whisk the seeds, egg whites, rosemary, pepper and salt together in a medium bowl. Pour egg mixture into skillet over vegetables. Cook at medium heat. Run a spatula around the bottom of the skillet as mixture sets, raising the mixture of eggs so that the uncooked part flows below. Continue cooking and edge lifting until the egg mixture is fully set, and the surface is only slightly moist.
3. Sprinkle with olives; cheese on top. Broil about 2 minutes or until the top is lightly browned and center is set. Let stand, before serving, for 5 minutes.

- Broccoli-cheddar quiche with a sweet potato crust

Ingredients

- 3 ¼ cups of sliced sweet potato (approx. 1 large)
- 1 large egg, lightly beaten
- 2 tablespoons of grated parmesan
- ¼ teaspoon of salt
- ⅛ teaspoon of pepper
- 2 cups of broccoli florets
- ¾ cup of grated cheddar cheese
- 3 tablespoons of chopped shallots
- 4 large eggs
- 1 tablespoon of sour cream
- 1 cup of low-fat milk
- ¼ teaspoon of salt
- ⅛ teaspoon of pepper

Preparation

1. Preheat oven to 400 degrees F to prepare the crust. Coat with cooking spray, a 9-inch deep-dish pie pan. In a medium bowl, whisk together sweet potato, 1 egg, Parmesan, 1/4 teaspoon salt and 1/8 teaspoon pepper. Move the mixture to the prepared pan and press it evenly to the bottom of the pan and to the sides. Bake for about 25 minutes, until the crust is set and begin to brown around the edges.
2. Evenly scatter broccoli, cheddar and shallots over the crust to prepare to fill and bake a quiche. In a small bowl, whisk eggs and sour cream, until

smooth. Whisk in milk, pepper and salt. Pour the egg mixture over the other ingredients for the filling. Reduce the Oven to 350 degrees F. Bake the quiche until the filling is in the center and start browning slightly, for 35 to 45 minutes. Until serving to allow to cool slightly.

- **Zucchini and oatmeal muffins**

Ingredient

- 1 tablespoon ground chia seeds
- 3 tablespoons of water
- 1 cup unsweetened almond milk
- 1 tablespoon lemon juice
- 1 teaspoon vanilla
- 1 cup gluten-free flour mix (for example, from the Trader Joe brand)
- ¾ cup gluten-free oatmeal (create yours by grinding oat flakes in the blender)
- ½ cup flaked gluten-free oatmeal
- ½ cup unprocessed or unrefined sugar (for example, Sucanat or turbinado)
- 2 teaspoons baking powder
- 1 teaspoon baking soda

- 1 teaspoon pumpkin pie spice
- ½ teaspoon of sea salt
- 1 ½ cups grated zucchini
- ½ cup raisins
- ½ cup walnuts, chopped

Preparations

1. Preheat the oven to 350 ° F (177 ° C)
2. Line a mold for 12 muffins with paper coverings.
3. In a small bowl, combine the ground chia seeds with water and let the mixture stand.
4. In a medium bowl, combine the almond milk with the lemon juice and let the mixture stand. Don't panic if it starts to set - you are supposed to!
5. Mix the flours, corn flakes, sugar, baking powder, baking soda, salt and pumpkin pie spice in a large bowl.
6. Add vanilla and chia seeds to the almond milk and lemon juice mixture and beat until everything is combined.
7. Add the wet ingredients to the dry ones and mix them until they are combined.
8. Add zucchini, raisins, and nuts. Let the dough rest for 5-10 minutes before filling the muffin pan.
9. Cook everyone from 21 to 23 minutes. Once the muffins have come out of the oven, wait 2-3 minutes before transferring them to the rack to cool them.

CHAPTER EIGHT
Mediterranean lunch recipes

- Garden fresh omelets

Ingredients

- 1 ⅓ cups of coarsely chopped tomatoes, drain
- 1 cup of roughly chopped, pitted cucumber
- Half a ripe avocado, halved, seeded, peeled and chopped
- ½ cup of roughly chopped red onion (1 medium)
- 1 clove of garlic, chopped
- Cut 2 tablespoons of fresh parsley
- 2 tablespoons of red wine vinegar
- 1 tablespoon of olive oil
- 2 eggs
- 1½ cups of chilled or frozen egg product, thawed
- ¼ cup of water
- 1 tablespoon of sliced fresh oregano or 1 teaspoon of dried oregano, crushed
- ¼ teaspoon of salt
- ¼ teaspoon of ground black pepper
- ⅛ teaspoon of crushed red pepper
- ¼ cup crumbled, reduced-fat feta cheese

Preparation

1. For salsa, stir tomatoes, cucumber, avocado, onion, garlic, parsley, vinegar and 1 teaspoon of oil together in a medium bowl.
2. Whisk the eggs, egg product, water, oregano, salt, black pepper together in a medium bowl and crush the red pepper. For each omelet, heat 1/2 teaspoon of the remaining oil over medium heat in an 8-inch non-stick skillet. Skillet with 1/2 cup of the egg mixture. Stir the eggs with a spatula until the mixture looks like fried bits of an egg surrounded by liquid. Stop stirring, but continue to cook until you set the egg. 1/3 cup of salsa spoon over one side of the egg mixture fried. Remove omelet from skillet; fold overfilling. Repeat to make a total of four omelets.
3. Serve per omelet with one-fourth of the salsa leftover. Sprinkle on 1 tablespoon of feta cheese with each omelet.

- Mediterranean chicken panini

Ingredients

- Olive oil non-stick cooking spray
- 2 small skinless, boneless chicken breasts (approx. 8 ounces in total)
- ⅓ cup of dried tomatoes (not oil-packed)

- 3 tablespoons of boiling water
- ⅓ Drain the cup of roasted red pepper in a bottle
- 4 teaspoons of balsamic vinegar
- 1 teaspoon of sliced fresh oregano or 1/2 teaspoon of dried oregano, crushed
- 1 large clove of garlic, chopped
- ⅛ teaspoon of ground black pepper
- 4 mini squares of wholemeal bagel bread or multigrain ciabatta rolls, divided
- 1 small zucchini

Preparations

1. Coat an unheated panini grid gently, covered indoor electric grill, or large non-stick skillet with non-stick spray cooking. Preheat to medium heat or heat, as regulated by the manufacturer. Stir in the chicken. Close the lid and grill for 6 to 7 minutes when using griddle or grill, or until chicken is no longer pink. (When using a skillet, cook chicken for 10 to 12 minutes or until chicken is no longer pink, turn once.) Cool the chicken slightly; divide each piece of chicken in half horizontally and cut into 2-inch wide slices crosswise.
2. Combine dried tomatoes with boiling water in a small pot. Cover and let 5 minutes stand. Transfer undrained tomato mixture to a small food processor (if you have a larger food processor, you will occasionally have to stop and scrape the sides

down). Attach roasted red sweet peppers, oregano, balsamic vinegar, big clove garlic, and ground black pepper. Cover and work smoothly before.

3. Place the dried tomato-pepper place over cut sides of squares of bagel bread. Place the chicken on the bread squares underneath. Cut very thin strips from the zucchini using a vegetable peeler. Layer slices of zucchini on top of the chicken. Place the tops of the square bagel on top of the zucchini, spread sides down. Click gently. Coat each sandwich lightly with nonstick cooking spray at the top and bottom.

4. Put sandwiches on board, grill, or skillet, if necessary attach in batches. Open the lid and grill for 2 to 3 minutes or until bread is toasted, if using griddle or grill. (If you use a skillet, place a heavy saucepan or skillet on top of the sandwiches. Cook for 1 to 2 minutes or until the bottoms are toasted. Carefully remove the saucepan or top skillet; it can be hot. Flip the sandwiches; cover with the saucepan or skillet again. Cook 1 to 2 minutes longer or until the bread is toasted.)

Spinach Stuffed Mushrooms

Ingredient

- 16 oz white whole mushrooms or "crimini."

- 3 crushed garlic cloves
- ¼ cup onion, minced
- ¼ cup white wine or vegetable stock
- 3 tablespoon low sodium soy sauce or tamari
- 3 cups sweet spinach
- ¼ cup white beans
- 2 tablespoons nutritional yeast
- ¼ red pepper, minced

Preparation

1. Preheat the oven to 375 degrees F.
2. Remove the stems from the mushrooms, leave the tops intact and chop the stems.
3. Sauté the onion, garlic, and mushroom stalks in a pan.
4. Add the wine and the soy sauce or tamari, continue cooking for 2-3 minutes, or until the vegetables soften a little.
5. Add the tender spinach and sauté for a minute.
6. move the vegetable mixture to a food processor.
7. Add beans and nutritional yeast and mix to combine.
8. Transfer to a bowl and mix the chopped red pepper.
9. Place the mushroom tops with the top side down in a baking dish.
10. Fill each mushroom top with the mixture.
11. Bake for 20-25 minutes.
12. Remove from oven and serve hot

Crispy Cauliflower Chips

Preparation

- Ahead of cauliflower, cut into florets
- ½ teaspoon garlic powder
- ½ teaspoon of seasoning for poultry or seasoning without salt (optional)
- ¾ cup of aquafaba
- 1 cup gluten-free bread crumbs

Preparation

1. Preheat the oven to 450 degrees F.
2. Put the cauliflower in a container and season with the garlic powder and the seasoning for birds (or without salt). Be sure to cover the cauliflower evenly.
3. Soak the cauliflower, a foil at once, in the aquafaba, and shake off the excess.
4. Cover with breadcrumbs and shake off excess.
5. Repeat with all cauliflower florets.
6. put the florets on a baking sheet lined with baking paper.
7. Bake for 15 minutes.
8. Turn the florets over to bake evenly.
9. Bake for another 15 minutes.

10. Serve immediately.

Baked potatoes without oil

Ingredient

- 4 medium yellow potatoes
- ½ teaspoon garlic powder
- sea salt and pepper to taste

preparations

1. Preheat the oven to 400 degrees F (218 degrees C).
2. Cut the potatoes into sticks similar to "fries" of approximately ½ "- ¾" thick.
3. Put the potatoes in a deep pot, cover with water, and boil for 5 minutes.
4. Drain well and pour it into a deep container.
5. Add the spices and cover the potatoes well with the seasoning.
6. Put the potatoes on a baking sheet covered with a silicone foil or baking paper.
7. Bake for 35-40 minutes or until cooked and crispy. Enjoy your meal!

- Red cranberry and kale pilaf

Ingredient

- 1 cup of brown rice
- 1 ¾ cups vegetable stock
- 1 small yellow onion, diced
- 12 ounces (340 grams) of kale (approximately 5 cups)
- 3 or 4 cloves garlic, minced
- ½ teaspoon red pepper flakes
- ½ cup dried cranberries
- ¼ cup chopped cashews or other nuts (optional)

Preparation

1. In a medium-sized pot or rice cooker, cook the rice in the broth according to package directions.
2. Sauté the onion for five minutes, or until it is transparent.
3. Add the kale (without stems and thickly chopped leaves) and cook for another five minutes, or until the kale is soft.
4. Add the garlic in flakes and red pepper and cook everything for another minute.
5. Add the cooked rice and continue sautéing for three minutes, or until the rice has completely warmed.
6. Remove the pan from the heat.
7. Add red cranberries and optional nuts, stir well.

- Sweet potato tropical casserole

Ingredient

- 4 cups diced sweet potatoes
- 1 cup diced mango
- 1 cup diced pineapple
- ½ teaspoon unsalted garlic and herb seasoning
- ½ cup pineapple and coconut juice

Process

1. Preheat oven to 350 degrees F.
2. Combine all ingredients in an 8 x 11 (2 qt) baking sheet.
3. Bake covered for 25 minutes.
4. Bake uncovered for 5 minutes and serve.

- Traditional stuffing

Ingredient

- ½ cup vegetable broth
- 1 spoon low sodium soy sauce or tamari
- 4 cups gluten-free or whole-wheat bread cubes
- ½ cup chopped onion
- 1 cup chopped celery
- 1 tablespoon nutritional yeast

- ½ teaspoon bird seasoning
- ½ teaspoon garlic powder
- ½ teaspoon dried parsley

Process

1. Preheat the oven to 350 F.
2. In a small bowl, mix the soil flax seeds with the water and set aside for 10 minutes.
3. In a big bowl, combine every dry ingredient.
4. Cut and place the apples in thin slices in a container.
5. Add the pumpkin puree, vanilla extract, water-based flaxseed, and apple date paste and blend well.
6. Combine the dry ingredients and blend well with the apples. If the mixture tends to be too dry, add water.
7. In an appropriate baking dish, put the mixture and bake for 30-35 minutes.

- **Quinoa Pilaf Stuffing**

Ingredient

- ½ teaspoon sage
- 1 teaspoon thyme
- 1 teaspoon rosemary
- ½ cup wild rice

- 1 ½ cups quinoa
- 1 cup brown rice or rice mix
- ½ cup freshly squeezed orange juice
- 2 ½ cups of vegetable stock
- ½ sea salt
- 1 cup grated carrots
- 1 cup pomegranate seeds (optional)
- 1 cup gooseberries (optional)

Process

1. Heat a pot over medium heat.
2. Add the spices to the pot and sauté for 30 seconds.
3. Add wild rice, quinoa, and brown rice and stir for 1 minute.
4. Add orange juice, vegetable broth, and sea salt, and stir well.
5. Bring to a boil, cover and reduce heat to medium-low and cook for 45 minutes.
6. Remove from heat, add carrots and fruit, and serve.

- Mashed sweet potato with cauliflower

Ingredient

- 1 head of cauliflower, without the core and cut into pieces

- 2 large sweet potatoes, peeled and cut into pieces of 1 inch (2.5 centimeters)
- ½ cup unsweetened vegetable milk
- 1 teaspoon garlic powder
- Salt and pepper to taste

Process

1. Steam the cauliflower and sweet potato in approximately 1-2 inches (2.5 - 5 centimeters) of water until soft. Alternatively, you can roast them on parchment paper in the oven at 400 ° F (204 ° C) for 20 to 30 minutes.
2. Add the soft vegetables to your food processor and process everything for one minute to dissolve the ingredients, or you can crush them by hand. Add the vegetable milk, garlic powder, salt, and pepper and continue processing until smooth.

- Brussels sprouts caramelized with blueberries.

Ingredient

- 8 chopped dates
- ½ cup of water
- 3 cups fresh Brussels sprouts, cut in half
- 1 cup fresh blueberries
- 1 tablespoon miso paste

- 1 cup low-sodium vegetable broth or water
- 1 organic red onion, chopped
- 1 tablespoon soy sauce
- ¼ cup of nuts such as almonds, Brazil nuts, several mixed, etc. (optional) Pepper to taste

Process

1. In a food processor, mix dates with ½ cup of water until a creamy texture is obtained. Set it aside for a moment.
2. In a saucepan over medium-high heat sauté the Brussels sprouts along with the onion, miso, blueberries and ½ cup of broth or water. Cook covered for 10 minutes or until lightly brown.
3. Stir frequently and add the rest of the additional liquid as necessary to prevent burning.
4. Cook the sprouts until they are caramelized by the edges.
5. Add the soy sauce, ground pepper, and date paste. Mix and match well.
6. Serve and garnish with nuts.

Mediterranean chicken with 4 kinds of cheese

Chicken breasts with tomato sauce with lemon peel and a variety of cheeses are served with screw noodles.

Ingredients

- 4 portions
- 4 halves boneless and skinless small breasts
- 1 can diced tomatoes
- 1/2 cup chopped black olives
- 1 tbsp grated lemon peel
- 1 cup five kinds of cheese finely, shredded, five cheese and blend
- In some supermarkets they all come in a bag

Steps

15 minutes

1. The breasts are fried in little oil for 7 minutes on each side, or until cooked.
2. Add the diced tomatoes, grated lemon peel and cook for 5 minutes.
3. This mixture is added to the chicken and it is taken to the fire for 2 minutes until everything has been well mixed, and finally the cheeses are put.
4. It is served with a screw paste and is also sprinkled with tomato sauce.

Mediterranean beef casserole

Ingredients

6 portions

- 900 gr aguayo steak (round steak palomilla) diced
- 2 tbsp Butter
- 1 can 340 grams of tomato paste
- 2/3 cup beef broth or red wine
- 1/2 cup sliced black olives
- 2 tbsp light brown light sugar
- 2 teeth chopped the garlic
- 1/4 cup red wine vinegar
- 2 leaves laurel
- 1/4 cup grapes
- 1 cdts ground cinnamon
- 1 cdts ground clove
- 3 cups hot steamed rice

process

50 minutes

- Preheat the oven to 375 F in a bowl, mix the steak, the melted butter settles in a baking dish.
- Mix in a bowl the tomato paste, the meat broth, the vinegar, add stirring the olives, sugar, garlic, pour over the steak. Turning it to spread it.

- Put the bay leaves on top of the meat mixture; distribute the raisins, cinnamon, cloves, cover with aluminum foil.
- Bake the casserole for 45 minutes, take out the bay leaves, discard them, arrange the cooked rice in a serving dish and on the rice, spread the meat and the sauce by spoonfuls.

Mediterranean rolls

Ingredients

4 portions

- 1 sliced eggplant
- 1 tbsp cheese
- 1 1/2 tbsp chia of
- 5 oz cream cheese
- 1/2 roasted pepper cut into brunoise
- 1cda post or fresh basil
- for in dressing:
- 1/2 tbsp white vinegar, olive oil to taste a touch of pesto
- salt and pepper to taste (the ingredients are mixed and olive oil is added in the form of thread until emulsified)

process

30 minutes

- The eggplant is cut into thin slices and grilled until softened.
- Mix the cheese, pepper, and basil, Parmesan cheese with mayonnaise mix everything, wrap this mixture with the eggplant slices and then add the dressing on top.
- Note: eggplants are put a decorative stick to hold. If you want you can take them to the oven but it is optional.

Mediterranean fish fillet

Ingredients

2 portions

- 2 steaks fish (Huauchinango, Robalo, Snapper, sea bream, etc.)
- 1-2 tomatoes
- 1 can mashed tomato
- black olives needed
- 1-2 teeth Garlic
- parsley

- Salt
- Pepper
- 1 Pope
- olive oil

process

30 minutes

- In a saucepan, we put olive oil and a clove of garlic chopped to brown when the aroma releases, add one or two peeled and chopped tomatoes, then add tomato puree, season with salt and pepper and add a peeled and diced potato 1 cm., we add some olives and chopped parsley. When the potatoes have been cooked, carefully place the fish fillets that are cooked over low heat, if necessary add a little water.
- Serve them with white rice.

Baked fish Mediterranean style

Ingredients

- 1 steak fish per person
- 3 chambray onions
- 1 tooth garlic for each steak
- red onion or échalots

- Salt
- Pepper
- dill powder
- olive oil
- Butter
- capers (optional)
- two lemons

process

20 minutes

- In a refractory we place our fish fillets on a little olive oil, and we put them on top: each: salt and pepper, a clove of minced garlic, chopped red onion or eschalots, the tails of about 3 small onions of chopped chambray and the onions are cut in half and placed on the sides, dill powder, a few capers, the juice of a lemon, olive oil and a piece of butter on top of each.
- It is put in a hot oven and you have to be on the lookout because it should not be more than 8 or 10 minutes so that it does not dry out, when we take it out we decorate the fillets with lemon slices.

Beef Meatballs in Vegetable Bath

Ingredients

6 portions

- 1/2 Bell pepper
- 1/2 stem celery
- 3 teeth natural garlic
- 3 teeth roasted garlic
- Chicken broth to liquefy the seasonings
- 4 ripe tomatoes
- 1 tbsp Mediterranean oil (canola-grape seeds-Extra virgin olive) to saute the seasoning
- 14 Large beef meatballs (baseball ball size)
- 16 oz of tomatoes in pieces with their juice
- 1 pinch ground turmeric
- 1 pinch ground cumin
- 1 tsp ground onion
- 16 ounces cooked and drained chickpeas
- Chicken broth as required.
- 1 cup carrots on thick wheels
- 6 pieces 1 baseball-size potato
- 1 cup peeled and chunky Aoyama

process

70 minutes

- Process the seasoning (the first 6 ingredients) and the tomatoes, in the blender covering with liquid chicken broth.
- In the pot you will prepare the broth, pour the oil and saute the liquefied seasoning.
- Add the meatballs, use pre-cooked and frozen. This speeds up the preparation process. Continue to soften and unite.
- Then add the carrot, chicken broth (I used broth prepared at home) but you can use the one you like. Add water to get the desired consistency. The Aoyama in pieces. Potatoes in large pieces. The can of tomato and the chickpeas drained.
- Add the Curcuma and cumin, after tasting taste.
- Reduce heat and cook until vegetables are tender.
- When extinguishing the fire add a sprig of thyme and oregano, preferably natural. Cover and let stand for 10 minutes before serving.
- It depends on the meat and personal taste, the fat is removed using a fat separator or allowing cooling because the fat floats on top and so you remove it.
- Accompany with white rice or bread

- Burritos of Cabbage

Ingredients

- One green or Chinese cabbage (12 leaves)
- 300 g ground beef
- One outing
- One clove of garlic
- 400 ml diced tomatoes
- One tablespoon tomato puree
- One tablespoon of taco herbs
- One small can of corn
- Two hands of grated cheese
- 100 gr kidney beans from a sack

Preparation

1. Chop the onion and then garlic and fry in a pan. Add the minced meat and then the taco herbs. Bake this loose. Stir in the tomato puree and cubes and then the drained corn and kidney beans. Let this burrito filling simmer for a few minutes. Meanwhile, boil water.
2. Heat the oven to 180 degrees. Cut the cabbage leaves and boil them (per 2 or 3) for a minute or 2 in the pan and then drain well. Place two cabbage leaves next to each other so that they overlap slightly. Spoon some of the burrito filling on one side, sprinkle with a little cheese and then carefully roll-up. Don't push too hard. Repeat this with the

rest of the cabbage leaves and filling. If they are all in the baking dish, sprinkle them with some extra cheese. Put the baking dish in the oven for about 15 minutes. Serve the carbohydrates with some rice (if the dish is no longer low in carbohydrates).

- Black Bean and Quinoa Burgers

Ingredient

- 3 cups cooked black beans
- 1 cup cooked quinoa
- 1 cup flaked oatmeal
- 2 tablespoons ground flaxseed
- ½ cup barbecue sauce
- ½ teaspoon of liquid smoke or smoked paprika
- 1 teaspoon garlic powder
- ½ teaspoon onion powder

Additional barbecue sauce for hamburger

Preparations

1. Preheat the oven to 400F.
2. Partially pest the beans.
3. include the rest of the ingredients and mix well.
4. Shape the burgers with your hands compacting well.

5. Put the burgers on a baking sheet covered with baking paper.
6. Bake the hamburgers for 15 minutes.
7. Flip the burgers and cover with a layer of barbecue sauce.
8. Bake for 10-15 more minutes.

Roasted Cauliflower with Turmeric

Ingredient

- 1 large cauliflower
- 2 teaspoons finely grated fresh ginger
- 1 tablespoon tahini
- 1 tablespoon organic miso paste, non-GMO
- 3 tablespoons vegetable stock
- 3 prunes or dates, chopped
- ½ teaspoon of turmeric powder
- 2 tablespoons tamari
- Ground black pepper, to taste
- Black and white sesame seeds, to decorate
- Sliced green onion, to decorate (optional)

Preparation

1. Preheat the oven to 425 degrees F.
2. Cut the leaves and stem at the bottom of the head of the cauliflower, so that it is flat.

3. Click with a sharp blade so that the spices penetrate the cauliflower.
4. Remove the cauliflower from the oven and sprinkle the top with one of the green onions (optional), the tamari, a pinch of ground black pepper, and sesame seeds before serving.
5. Mix the ginger, tahini, miso paste, broth, prums or dates, and turmeric in a food processor.
6. Rub the paste over the cauliflower using your hands, ensuring that it is spread everywhere, even at the edges.
7. In the oven, roast the cauliflower for 45 minutes or until golden is soft and cool.

- Creamy mushroom lasagna, gluten-free

Ingredient

- 3 cloves garlic, ground
- 16 ounces of chopped champignons (you can use a mixture of different champignons)
- 1 tablespoon of tamari or aminos (amino acids in liquid, in Spanish) of coconut or soy sauce, gluten-free
- 1 teaspoon dried thyme
- Thirty-four cup raw cashews, soaked for a few hours, drained overnight.

- 1 cup vegetable broth + a little more to saute garlic and mushrooms
- 2 large handfuls of spinach
- 10 ounces of lasagna sheets, gluten-free (I love Tinkyada brown rice pasta)
- 4 cups marinara sauce, purchased at the store (a 32 oz or 946 ml bottle) or homemade
- Nutritional Yeast (optional)

Preparations

1. In a skillet, heat a little vegetable stock at medium temperature. When it is hot, add the garlic and skip it until it releases the aroma. This will take a minute. Add the mushrooms, tamari (or coconut or soy amino sauce, gluten-free), and thyme. Cook, mix more or less every minute, for six or eight minutes or until the mushrooms release their water, and a small broth begins to form.
2. Combine cashews and vegetable broth in a high-speed blender and blend until the mixture is completely uniform. This may take five minutes, depending on your blender's speed and power. Verse the cashew sauce with the mushrooms in the pan. Reduce heat to medium-low and simmer to let the sauce thicken, stirring frequently.
3. make the lasagna sheets according to the package instructions. Be sure to do this after your mushroom sauce is ready so that the slices do not remain static

for a long time and begin to stick. Spread a third of the marinara sauce in the bottom of a baking sheet eight to eleven inches in size (20 to 28 cm). Add a layer of sheets. Cover them with half the mushroom cream. Add a layer of sheets. Use another third of the marinara sauce to cover them. Add the remaining mushroom cream. Add the last layer of sheets and cover them with the remaining marinara sauce.

4. Cover the lasagna with foil and bake for 30 minutes. Remove the paper, add some nutritional yeast on top, if you want, and cook it for another 15 minutes. Let the lasagna stand for five minutes before serving.

Traditional Greek salad

Ingredients

- 2 tomatoes
- Cucumber
- 3 small red onions
- A handful of green and black olives
- 25 dag feta
- 2-3 tablespoons of wine vinegar
- 6 tablespoons olive oil

- 2 tablespoons oregano
- Salt
- pepper

How to prepare the recipe:

1. Peel cucumbers and onions, wash tomatoes. Dice tomatoes and cucumbers, and onions into rings. Mix the vegetables . Cut the feta

into cubes, add to vegetables along with olives.

2. We prepare the sauce: mix the oil with wine vinegar, season with salt and pepper. We pour the salad. We sprinkle with oregano.

Tomato and feta salad

Ingredients

- 2 tablespoons of balsamic vinegar
- 1/ 2 teaspoons of chopped fresh basil or 1/2 teaspoon of dried basil
- 1/2 teaspoon of salt
- 1/2 cup of roughly chopped sweet onion
- 1 pound grape or cherry tomatoes, halved
- 2 tablespoons of olive oil
- 1/4 cup crumbled feta cheese

Directions

1. Mix vinegar, basil and salt in a large bowl. Add onion; throw to coat. Let it rest for 5 minutes. Add the tomatoes, oil and feta; throw to coat. Serve with a slotted spoon.

Colorful layered salad

Ingredients

- iceberg lettuce
- tomatoes
- ¾ cans of corn
- medium cucumbers
- yellow pepper
- 2-3 red onions
- chicken breasts (about 0.5 kg)
- seasoning for peas and chicken
- 2-3 pieces of bread
- seasoning for toasts
- Butter and oil for frying
- Herb sauce

How to prepare the recipe:

1. Cut the chicken into small pieces, sprinkle with gyros and chicken, the season in the fridge for 1-2 hours.
2. Layer the salad in layers. We tear the lettuce and put the dishes on the bottom. Cut the tomatoes into halves or slices. We drain the corn. Peel cucumbers and cut into halves or slices. Then cut the peppers into strips. Cut the red onions into quarters of the slices.
3. We heat oil and fry chicken.
4. Cut the bread into small cubes, warm up the butter in a pan and pour the sliced bread on them. Fry until golden brown, sprinkle with a toast to the end of frying.
5. We prepare herbal sauce according to the recipe on the packaging and pour the whole salad before serving.

- **Nopal Soup**

What you will need

- 2 pounds of nopales, clean and diced
- 4 Roma tomatoes
- ¼ white onion
- 2 cloves of garlic

- 1 chipotle chili in adobo (optional)
- 3 cups of vegetable stock
- 1 tablespoon dried oregano
- Salt and pepper to taste

OPTIONAL COVERAGES

- Avocado
- Coriander
- Chives
- Lemon or Lime Juice

Preparation

1. Cook the nopales for 20-25 minutes in boiling water with salt or until they lose their bright color and are tender to bit.
2. Place the tomatoes, onion, garlic, and chipotle in a blender glass. Blend until you get a creamy consistency.
3. Remove the nopales from the heat, drain them, and rinse them with enough cold water. Leave aside.
4. In a pot, sauté the tomato sauce for about 3 minutes.
5. Add cooked nopales and oregano to tomato broth. Let cook another 15 minutes.
6. add salt and pepper to taste.
7. Serve on soup plates and add toppings.

- Matzo Ball Soup

What you will need

MATZO BALLS

- 1 ½ cups quinoa flakes
- 1 ½ cups of mixture gluten purpose flour
- 2 teaspoons onion powder
- 1 teaspoon garlic powder
- ¼ teaspoon of sea salt
- 2 cups of boiling water
- 6 tablespoons pumpkin puree

SOUP

- 1 medium yellow onion, chopped
- ¼ cup of Coconut Aminos
- ½ teaspoon freshly ground black pepper
- 5 medium carrots, peeled and sliced
- 3 celery stalks, diced
- 2 parsnips, peeled and sliced
- 1 cup fresh parsley, chopped
- 8 cups of vegetable broth without sodium

COVER

- 3 tablespoons fresh dill, finely chopped

Preparation

1. Preheat the oven to 200-300 degrees F (148 ° C). Cover a 15 x 13 inch (38 x 33 cm) baking sheet with parchment paper.
2. To make matzo balls: Beat quinoa flakes, flour, onion powder, garlic powder, and salt in a medium bowl. Add the boiling water and the pumpkin and stir to combine.
3. Take at least a tablespoon of the mixture and form a ball. Place the ball on the prepared baking sheet. Repeat until you have used the entire mixture. You should have approximately 30 balls.
4. Bake the matzo balls until they are a light golden color, approximately 20 minutes. Turn the balls halfway through cooking.
5. Transfer the baking sheet from the oven to a wire rack and let it stand for 10 minutes.
6. To make the soup: heat the onion in a large pot over medium heat and stir until it begins to release its aroma, approximately for a minute.
7. Add the Coconut Aminos, black pepper, carrots, celery, parsnips, and parsley and cook, stirring occasionally, until the vegetables release their aroma and are slightly soft, about two minutes. Add the broth and boil.
8. Reduce the heat intensity, cover the pot, and let simmer for about 35 minutes.
9. Serve immediately and place several matzo balls in each bowl of soup. Sprinkle dill in the soup.

10. The soup tastes even better the next day, and even better two days later.

CHAPTER NINE
Mediterranean dinner recipes

- Mediterranean Baked Cod Recipe with Lemon and Garlic

Ingredients

- 1.5-pound cod fillet pieces (4-6 pieces)
- 5 garlic cloves, peeled and minced
- 1/4 cup chopped fresh parsley leaves
- 5 tablespoons of fresh lemon juice
- 5 tablespoons of private extra virgin olive oil
- tablespoons of melted butter
- 1/3 cup all-purpose flour
- 1 teaspoon of coriander powder
- 3/4 teaspoons of Spanish sweet pepper
- 3/4 teaspoon ground cumin
- 3/4 teaspoons of salt
- 1/2 teaspoon black pepper

Preparation

1. Preheat the oven to 400 F.
2. In a shallow bowl, combine the lemon juice, olive oil and melted butter. Set aside Mix flour, spices, salt and pepper for all uses in another shallow bowl. Put the mixture next to the lemon juice.

3. Dry fish fillet with pat. Dip the fish in a lemon juice mixture, then dip it in a flour mixture. Shake off excess flour.
4. Heat 2 tablespoons of olive oil over medium-high heat in a cast-iron skillet (look at the oil to make sure it is sizzling but not smoky). Add fish and sear on each side to give it some color, but don't cook completely (about a few minutes on each side) Remove from heat.
5. Attach the minced garlic to the remaining lemon juice mixture and blend. Drizzle the fish fillets all over.
6. Bake until it starts to flake easily with a fork in the heated oven (10 minutes should be finished, but start checking earlier). Remove the chopped parsley from heat and sprinkle with it.
7. Serving suggestions: Serve with Lebanese rice and this Mediterranean chickpea salad or the popular Greek immediately

- Chicken Shawarma

Ingredients

- 3/4 tablespoons ground cumin
- 3/4 tablespoons of turmeric powder
- 3/4 tablespoons of coriander powder
- 3/4 tablespoons of garlic powder
- 3/4 tablespoons of paprika

- 1/2 teaspoon of ground cloves
- 1/2 teaspoon cayenne pepper, more if you prefer
- salt
- boneless and skinless chicken legs
- 1 large onion, thinly sliced
- 1 large lemon, juice of
- 1/3 cup private extra virgin olive oil reserve
- 6 pita pockets
- Tahini sauce or Greek tzatziki sauce
- rocket salad
- ingredients of Mediterranean salad
- Pickled olives or Kalamata (optional)

Preparation

1. Mix the cumin, turmeric, coriander, garlic powder, sweet paprika and cloves together in a small bowl. Place the shawarma spice blend aside for now.
2. Pat the chicken thighs on both sides, dry and season with salt, then slice thinly into small pieces of bite-size.
3. Place the chicken inside a big bowl. Remove the spices of shwarma, and toss to coat. Add the onions, the juice of the lemon and the butter. Again throw all together. Cover and cool for 3 hours or overnight (if you have no time, you can cut or miss the marinating time)
4. Preheat the oven to 425 degrees F when they are ready. Take out the chicken from the fridge and let it sit for a few minutes at room temperature.

5. Spread the marinated chicken over a large, lightly oiled baking sheet pan with the onions in one layer. Roast the 425 degrees F heated-oven for 30 minutes. Moves the pan to the top rack and broil very quickly (watch carefully) for a more browned, crispier chicken. Remove from the frying pan.
6. Prepare the pita pockets whilst the chicken roasts. Create tahini sauce as per this recipe, or Tzatziki sauce as per this recipe. Create the Mediterranean salad3-ingredient according to this recipe. Deposit aside.
7. Open the pita pockets, to eat. Spread a little tahini or tzatziki sauce, add chicken shawarma, arugula, Mediterranean salad and, if you like, pickles or olives. Eat straight away!

- Moroccan vegetable tagine recipe

Ingredients

- 1/4 cup of Riserva extra virgin olive oil, more for later
- medium yellow onions, peeled and chopped
- 8-10 cloves of garlic, peeled and chopped
- large carrots, peeled and chopped
- 2 large red potatoes, peeled and diced
- 1 large sweet potato, peeled and diced
- sale

- 1 tablespoon of a mixture of Harissa species
- 1 tablespoon of coriander powder
- 1 teaspoon ground cinnamon
- 1/2 teaspoon turmeric powder
- 2 cups canned whole peeled tomatoes
- 1/2 cup chopped dried apricot
- 1 liter of low sodium vegetable broth (or broth of your choice)
- 2 days of cooked chickpeas
- 1 lime, juice of
- A handful of fresco parsley leaves

Preparation

1. Heat olive oil over medium heat in a large heavy bowl, or Dutch Oven, until shimmering. Add the onions, and heat up to medium-high. Saute for 5 minutes, tossing periodically.
2. Remove all the chopped veggies and the garlic. Season with herbs and salt. Toss to merge.
3. Cook on medium-high heat for 5 to 7 minutes, and mix frequently with a wooden spoon.
4. Garnish with onions, apricot and broth. Spice with a slight dash of salt once more.
5. Keep over medium-high heat, and cook for 10 minutes. Reduce heat, cover and simmer for another 20 to 25 minutes or tender before veggies.
6. Stir in chickpeas and cook over low heat for another 5 minutes.

7. Incorporate lemon juice, and fresh parsley. Seasoning to taste and change, adding more salt or harissa spice mix to your liking.
8. Move to bowls for serving and finish each with a generous drizzle of extra virgin olive oil from Private Reserve. Serve hot with couscous, or pasta, your favorite meal.

- **Green salad with Chicken Rey and egg**

Ingredients

- 1/2 iceberg lettuce
- 2 carrots
- 2 hard-boiled eggs
- 1 chicken breast
- 1 tomato
- Mayonnaise
- olive oil
- Pepper
- Salt

Preparation

- Wash and cut the iceberg lettuce to Juliana. We booked in a large bowl.

- We wash and cut the tomato into dice. We add to the bowl.
- Peel and cut the carrot julienne. We add to the bowl.
- Cut the chicken breast into strips.
- Cook the eggs for 10-15 minutes in a saucepan with a stream of vinegar and salt, so that they do not break.
- When the eggs are ready, we remove, cool with a jet of water and remove the shell.
- Chop the hard-boiled eggs into quarters and add to the bowl.
- Meanwhile in a pan with a drizzle of oil, place the chicken strips, season and brown the chicken for 5 minutes over medium heat.
- Mix the salad with a couple of tablespoons of mayonnaise to taste and serve immediately.

- Panera Bread Green Goddess Cobb Salad

Ingredients

Pickled onions:

- 1 cup of sliced red onion
- 1/2 cup white vinegar
- 1 tablespoon of sugar

- 1 1/2 teaspoon of salt
- 1 cup of warm water

Salad servers:

- 6 ounces of salad mix-use rocket, romaine, kale, and radicchio mix
- 6 ounces of grilled chicken breast
- 2 tablespoons of crispy cooked bacon
- 3 tablespoons of chopped avocado
- 1/2 cup of chopped tomatoes
- Halve 1 hard-boiled egg
- 2 tablespoons of feta
- 2 tablespoons of pickled onions

Green goddess salad dressing:

- 1 cup of mayonnaise
- 2 tablespoons of tarragon leaves
- 3 tablespoons of chopped chives
- 1 cup of flat-leaf parsley
- 1 cup of packed watercress cleaned and hard stems removed
- 2 tablespoons of lemon juice
- 1 tablespoon of champagne vinegar
- 1/2 teaspoon of salt
- 1/4 teaspoon of pepper

Direction

- Cut onions as thin as possible, I like to use the 1/8 inch setting on my mandolin. Put the onions in a jar wide. Mix white vinegar, sugar, salt and warm water in a small bowl. Stir until sugar and salt have dissolved. These should rest for about 30 minutes for use.
- Put all the ingredients for the dressing in the bowl of a blender or food processor and mix for 30-45 seconds, or until the dressing is mostly smooth and creamy.
- Place the salad on the bottom of a large salad bowl. Cut the chicken breast into thin slices and place on the salad. Add bacon, chopped avocado, chopped tomatoes, feta cheese, hard-boiled egg halves, and pickled onions. Drizzle with as much salad dressing as desired. Remaining salad dressing can be kept in an airtight container for 1 week.
- Caprese tomato, mozzarella, basil and avocado salad recipe

Ingredients

- 2 sliced avocados
- 2 ripe tomatoes
- 500 g mozzarella cheese
- 1 cup fresh basil leaves
- 1/4 cup olive oil
- 1/4 cup balsamic Aceto

- Salt and ground black pepper

Direction

- Gather all the ingredients to make this tomato, mozzarella, basil, and avocado Caprese salad.
- With a small knife, cut the end of the tomato stem and then, using a serrated knife, cut the tomatoes into slices.
- Cut the mozzarella into slices and see alternating slices of avocado, tomato, mozzarella and basil leaves in individual dishes.
- Sprinkle with olive oil and balsamic vinegar and season lightly with salt and ground black pepper.
- Spread your Italian tomato, mozzarella, basil and avocado salad with a fresh baguette or on a bed of romaine lettuce.

- Creamy Potato Salad

Ingredients

- 1 kilo of potatoes
- ¾ cups of low-fat sour cream
- ¼ cup of mayonnaise
- ¼ cup chopped fresh parsley
- 3 tablespoons lemon juice
- 2 tablespoons Dijon mustard

- 2 tablespoons chopped fresh tarragon
- 2 chopped celery stalks
- 2 hard-boiled eggs
- 1 small fennel, thinly sliced

Direction

- Peel the potatoes and cut them into medium cubes. Place them in a large pot with cold water and kosher salt to taste, and add a little salt. Bring to the fire and when it boils, simmer until the potatoes are tender 10 to 12 minutes.
- Mix mayonnaise with sour cream, mustard and lemon juice.
- Season with salt and ground black pepper and add warm potatoes. Mix and let cool to room temperature.
- Add the celery cut into thin slices as well as fennel and parsley and tarragon, all finely chopped.
- Mix so that the potatoes are impregnated with cream and add the hard-cut eggs in wedges. Serve the creamy potato salad.

- Wedge Salad with Creamy Dressing

Ingredients

- 1 cup Daisy Cream

- 1/2 cup skim milk
- 4 teaspoons cider vinegar
- 1 sachet of green onion powder mix
- 1 clove garlic, minced
- 1/2 cup sliced green onion
- 1 head of iceberg lettuce, removed the heart and in pictures
- 1 tomato, diced
- 4 teaspoons diced bacon

Instructions

- In a small bowl, combine the cream, buttermilk, vinegar and dressing mix. Beat until the mixture is smooth. Add garlic and 1/4 cup green onion; set aside. Remove the center of the lettuce and cut into 4 equal wedges. Place each wedge in four different dishes. Pour about 1/4 of the salad dressing over each wedge. Distribute 1/4 of the remaining onion, 1/4 of the chopped tomato and 1 teaspoon of diced bacon on top of each wedge.

- Tomatoes stuffed with tuna

Ingredients

- 2 cans of water or natural tuna
- 4 medium tomatoes
- 1 large cup of white or brown rice
- Mayonnaise c / n
- Green olives c / n
- Peas or capers c / n
- 2 carrots
- Salt c / n

Direction

- Place plenty of water in a pot and bring it to the fire. When it boils, pour the rice. Stir with a wooden spoon so that it does not stick and cook for 20 minutes or until it is soft. Remove, drain immediately and reserve in the fridge.
- Peel the carrots and cut them into small cubes. Cook in a pot with water until they soften. Drain and place in a bowl.
- Add the rice, the two cans of drained tuna, the peas or capers (cooked) and the mayonnaise to taste.
- Mix everything very well and room to taste.
- Wash the tomatoes very well and smoke them with the help of a knife and a spoon.
- If you want to take advantage of what you have taken to the tomato, cut it into small cubes and mix it with the rice or reserve it for another recipe.

- Fill the tomatoes with the rice and the tuna. Garnish with some mayonnaise in the center and a green olive.

Seafood paella recipe

Ingredients

- 4 small lobster tails (6-12 ounces each)
- water
- tablespoons of extra virgin olive oil from the reserve
- 1 large yellow onion, chopped
- cups of Spanish rice or medium-grain rice, soaked in water for 15-20 minutes and then drained
- garlic cloves, minced
- 2 large pinches of Spanish saffron threads, dipped in 1/2 cup of water
- 1 teaspoon Spanish sweet pepper
- 1 teaspoon cayenne pepper
- 1/2 teaspoon of Aleppo pepper flakes
- salt
- 2 large Roma tomatoes, finely chopped
- ounces of green beans, cut
- 1 kilo of prawns or large prawns or your choice, peeled and gutted
- 1/4 cup chopped fresh parsley

Preparation

1. Take about 3 cups of water in a large pot to a rolling boil. Attach the lobster tails and let boil until pink for a very brief time (1-2 minutes). Then turn off the heat. Attach a pair of tongs to the lobster tails. Do not waste cooking water on the lobster. When the lobster is sufficiently cool for handling, remove the shell and break it into large chunks.
2. Heat 3 tbsp of olive oil in a large deep pan, or cast-iron skillet. Turn the heat and add the chopped onions to medium-high. Saute the onions for 2 minutes then add the rice, and cook 3 minutes more, stirring frequently. Now add cooking water for the chopped garlic and the lobster. Extract the saffron and the oil, paprika, cayenne pepper, Aleppo pepper and salt are soaking. Attach the chopped tomato and green beans. Bring to a boil and let the liquid reduce slightly, then cover (with a lid or tightly with foil) and cook for 20 minutes at low heat.
3. Uncover and scatter the shrimp over the rice, gently pressing it into the water. Add some water, if necessary. Cover for another 10 minutes and cook until the shrimp turns pink. Finally add bits of fried lobster. Turn heat off when the lobster gets warmed up. Garnish with peregrinate.
4. Serve the delicious paella with your white wine of choice.

- Spaghetti and Meatballs

Ingredient

- 1½ cup of water
- ¾ cup of millet
- 1 small yellow onion, finely diced
- 4 cloves garlic, ground
- 1 tablespoon dried basil
- 1 teaspoon ground fennel seeds
- 1 teaspoon red pepper crushed flakes (optional)
- ¼ cup dried tomatoes, finely chopped
- ¼ cup artichoke hearts, finely chopped
- ¼ cup roasted pine nuts or walnuts, chopped into large pieces
- 1 teaspoon sea salt (optional)
- 1 pound whole-grain cereal spaghetti
- 1 jar (28 ounces or 828 ml) hot spaghetti sauce
- Fresh chopped parsley, for decorat

Preparation

1   Preheat the oven to 375 ° F (191 ° C).

2. To make the meatballs, combine the water and millet in a small saucepan and bring the water to a boil at high temperature. Reduce it to medium-low and cook the millet until it is tender about 20 minutes. If it is not tender after all the water is absorbed, add two or three tablespoons of water and let it cook for another five minutes.
3. While the millet is cooking, sauté the onion in a large skillet at medium-high temperature until it becomes translucent and begins to brown, approximately for five minutes. Add the garlic, basil, fennel, and red pepper flakes (if you use it) and cook for another minute. Add dried tomatoes, artichoke hearts, and nuts (if you use them) and remove the pan from the heat.
4. When the millet is ready, add it to the pan with the onion mixture, add the sea salt (if you use it) and mix well. Shape the mixture into balls using an ice cream spoon or a 1/3 cup measure and place them on nonstick baking paper.
5. Bake for like 15 minutes, turn them over and continue baking until the millet balls are lightly browned, about 15 minutes more.
6. To make the spaghetti while the meatballs are baking, cook the spaghetti according to the package instructions and drain it.

7. Transfer the cooked spaghetti to a larger tray. Top with meatballs and spaghetti sauce. Garnish with parsley and serve.

Oatmeal Seasoned with Vegetables

Ingredient

- 4 cups of water
- 2 cups of "cut" oatmeal (quick-cooking steel-cut oats)
- 1 teaspoon Italian spices
- ½ teaspoon Herbamare or sea salt
- 1 teaspoon garlic powder
- 1 teaspoon onion powder
- ½ cup nutritional yeast
- ¼ teaspoon turmeric powder
- 1½ cup kale or tender spinach
- ½ cup sliced mushrooms
- ¼ cup grated carrots
- ½ cup small chopped peppers

Preparation

1. Boil the water in a saucepan.
2. Add the oatmeal and spices and lower the temperature.
3. Cook over low heat without lid for 5 to 7 minutes.

4. Add the vegetables.
5. Cover and set aside for 2 minutes.
6. Serve immediately.

Rice with Smoked Sausages and Beer

Ingredients

- 14 smoked beef sausage
- 3 1/2 cups raw rice
- 1/2 onion in small cubes
- 1/2 chili pepper in small cubes
- 1 tbsp crushed garlic
- 1 cube chicken soup
- 1/4 cup tomato sauce
- water to prepare rice
- 1 tbsp Mediterranean oil (olive-canola-grapeseed)

Preparation

1. You add the oil to the pot you use; personally I prefer the quick pot for your convenience. Heat over medium heat; add the onion, bell pepper, and garlic, sauté, joining well.
2. Add the sausages, continue sautéing until they have browned the tomato sauce, and continue joining.

3. Rub the beer stream and continue joining while you jump. And you allow the alcohol to evaporate,
4. The rice, mix well and sauté for about 1 minute.
5. Add enough water to prepare the rice; this will depend on the pot you are using.
6. try salt and cook like normal rice

CHAPTER TEN
Mediterranean dessert recipes

- Italian apple and olive oil cake

Ingredients

- large gala apples, peeled and chopped as finely as possible
- Orange juice for soaking apples
- cups of all-purpose flour
- 1/2 teaspoon ground cinnamon
- 1/2 teaspoon ground nutmeg
- 1 teaspoon of baking powder
- 1 teaspoon of baking powder
- 1 cup of sugar
- 1 cup of private extra virgin olive oil
- 2 large eggs
- 2/3 cup of golden raisins, immersed in hot water for 15 minutes and then draining well
- Icing sugar for dusting

Preparations

1. Oven preheats to 350 degrees F.
2. In a cup, place the sliced apples, and add the orange juice. Just enough juice to throw in the apples and clean them so they don't shine.

3. Sift the flour, cinnamon, nutmeg, baking powder and baking powder into a large bowl. Add the sugar and extra virgin olive oil to a blender bowl with whisk for now. Remove at low temperature for 2 minutes, until all is well mixed

4. Add the eggs one by one with the mixer on and stir for another 2 minutes, until the mixture volume increases (it should be denser but still fluid).

5. With the dry ingredients in the large bowl, indent in the center of the flour mixture. Pour the wet mixture into the well (mix of sugar and olive oil). Replace with a wooden spoon until all have blended properly. It will be a thick batter (let nothing be added to loosen this).

6. Let the raisins dry absolutely soak in the bowl. And rid the excess juice of the apples. Add the raisins and apples to the batter and stir until all is well mixed with a spoon. The dough is going to be quite dense again.

7. Layer a 9-inch parchment paper cake saucepan. In the pan put a thick batter and align the top with the wooden spoon back.

8. Bake for 45 minutes at 350 ° F, or until a toothpick or wooden skewer has been inserted.

9. Keep it in the pan to cool completely. Just raise the parchment when you're done to put the cake in a tub. The powder was containing icing sugar. Alternatively heat up some dark honey (those with a sweeter tooth like this option) to serve.

Chocolate Panna Cotta

Ingredient

- Half a liter of special liquid cream to assemble
- 100 ml of milk
- 1 tablet of chocolate for desserts (black or milk, to your liking) of 100 gr
- A splash (25 ml) of Grand Marnier or an orange liqueur
- 100 gr of sugar (or something less, it depends on the sweetness of chocolate and your tastes)
- 6 sheets of neutral jelly or 1 sachet of powdered gelatin (10 gr)

Preparation

1. Melt the chocolate in a water bath or in the microwave at medium power for about 5 min. We hydrate the gelatin leaves in a little water (about 10-15 min are enough).
2. Mix the cream with the melted chocolate over the heat and add the sugar, milk, and liquor, beating well so that the sugar dissolves. We must avoid getting to boil and we must not stop stirring so that lumps do not

form. We also incorporate the gelatin and continue stirring until it dissolves well.
3. We fill some molds with this cream and leave in the fridge a few hours until it sets. I usually use individual silicone molds because it is easier to unmold and I like this candy more individually.

Drunk chocolate cake with mousse and strawberries

Ingredient

- 3 cups all-purpose gluten-free flour
- ½ cup date or coconut sugar
- 2 teaspoons baking powder
- 1 teaspoon baking soda
- ½ teaspoon of sea salt
- 6 tablespoons cocoa powder
- 4 tablespoons ground flax seeds
- 4 teaspoons vanilla extract
- 4 tablespoons unsweetened applesauce
- 2 tablespoons apple cider vinegar
- 1 cup raisins
- 2 cups of cold water

COVERAGES

- 8 cups fresh or thawed strawberries

- 4 cups of chocolate mousse

Preparation

1. Preheat the oven to 350 degrees F.
2. In a large container, combine flour, sugar, baking powder, baking soda, cocoa powder, ground flaxseed (flax), and salt.
3. In a blender, mix the water and raisins well.
4. Pour the raisin water mixture into a separate bowl and combine it with the vinegar, vanilla, and applesauce.
5. Pour the wet ingredients over the dry ones and stir with a whisk until well mixed.
6. Pour the mixture into a round baking dish covered with baking paper.
7. Bake for 30 minutes.
8. Remove from the oven and wait for it to cool.
9. To assemble the drunk cake, start by spreading a layer of chocolate mousse at the bottom of a cake pie bowl, a round bowl, or a cup of personal size parfait.
10. Cover the mousse with a layer of strawberries.
11. Place a layer of cake. If you opt for a personal parfait, you can use a round cookie cutter to cut the cake.
12. Repeat steps 9-11 until you fill the bowl or cup.
13. The last layer should be chocolate and strawberry mousse.

- crunchy quinoa bars

Ingredients

- 4-ounce semi-sweet chocolate bars
- 1 cup of dry quinoa
- 1 tablespoon of PB2
- 1/2 teaspoon vanilla
- For the peanut butter dressing:
- spoons of water
- 1/2 tablespoons of PB2

Preparation

1. Heat a pan with a heavy bottom over medium to high heat. Let it warm up for a couple of minutes before adding some quinoa Add 1/4 cup quinoa at once (so you'll have four batches to pop). Let it rest on the bottom of the pot, turning occasionally, until you start hearing the crackling of light, then constantly shake it for about a minute, until the explosion has slightly subsided. Be sure to take it off before it turns brown (it can happen very fast). You don't want anything but a toasted golden color Once all of your quinoa has sprouted, place it aside in a small bowl.
2. In a bowl, add the melted chocolate, quinoa, PB2 and vanilla-mix to thoroughly combine Line a baking sheet with parchment paper and spread your chocolate quinoa mixture on top: you do NOT have to scatter the

mixture over the whole pan, or it will be too thin. Just the middle form a square shape. The thickness is up to you - but in a small bowl, I made mine about 1/2 inch thick, add the peanut butter drizzle together. Sprinkle it all over the top of the chocolate and quinoa, then use a knife to shake it gently Refrigerate for at least one hour before slicing (or until it's absolutely hard). When sliced, I keep mine in the fridge, but the counter still works!

- Apple and pumpkin pie

Ingredient

- 1 spoon ground flax seeds + 2 ½ tablespoons water (flax egg)
- ½ cup all-purpose gluten-free flour (or oatmeal)
- 1 ½ cup quick-cooking oatmeal
- 1 tablespoon baking powder
- 1 teaspoon baking soda
- 2 tablespoons pumpkin pie spice
- 1 tablespoon cinnamon
- 4 medium granny smith apples
- ½ cup date pasta
- 1 cup pumpkin puree
- 1 teaspoon vanilla extract
- ¼ cup of water (optional)

Preparations

1. Preheat the oven to 350 degrees F.
2. Mix ground flaxseed (flax) seeds with water in a small bowl and set aside for 10 minutes.
3. Mix all dry ingredients in a large bowl.
4. Cut the apples into thin slices and place them in a container.
5. Add the pumpkin puree, vanilla extract, flaxseed with water, and date paste to apples and mix well.
6. merge the dry ingredients with the apples and mix well. Add water if the mixture seems to be too dry.
7. Place the mixture in an 8 x 11 (2 quarts) container suitable for baking and bake for 30-35 minutes.

- **Blueberry muffins**

Recipe

Dough

- 28 g coconut flour
- 56 g butter (melted)
- 56 g of erythritol
- 3 eggs
- 5 tbsp whipped blueberries
- 1 tsp vanilla extract
- 1/2 tsp baking powder

- 1/4 tsp salt

Topping

- 113 g cream cheese (softened)
- 56 g butter (softened)
- 5 tbsp whipped blueberries
- 1 tbsp erythritis
- 1/2 tsp vanilla extract

Cooking

Dough

1. Combine butter, eggs, erythritol, and vanilla extract.
2. Add coconut flour, baking powder, and salt. Beat until smooth.
3. Add the blueberry mixture and mix thoroughly.
4. Pour the batter into the muffin pan.
5. Bake for 30 minutes at 200 degrees.
6. Remove from the oven and cool.

- Brownie Fat Bombs

Ingredients

- 110 g soft unsalted butter
- 30 g soft cream cheese
- 3 tbsp melted coconut oil

- ½ cup almond flour
- ⅓ cup of powdered keto sweetener to your taste
- ¼ cup unsweetened cocoa powder
- 1 tsp vanilla essence
- ⅓ cups of crushed chocolate without sugar (minimum 80% cocoa)

Cooking

1. Put butter, cream cheese, and coconut oil in a bowl. Beat with a mixer until smooth.
2. Add almond flour, sweetener, cocoa powder and vanilla essence. Beat well until smooth.
3. Add chocolate and mix.
4. Cool the mixture for 1 hour or until solid.
5. Form balls the size of a tablespoon and place on a baking sheet with parchment.
6. Cool the balls for another 30 minutes before storing them in an airtight container in the refrigerator or freezer.

- chocolate Custard

Ingredients

- 310 ml unsweetened almond milk

- 310 ml oily whipped cream
- 6 egg yolks
- ⅓ cup stevia or erythritis
- 2 tsp vanilla essence
- 225 g sugar-free chocolate chips

Cooking

1. Add all ingredients except chocolate and whipped cream to the pan. Beat well.
2. Put on low heat and stir continuously for 15 minutes until the mixture thickens.
3. Add the chocolate and mix well until all the chocolate has melted and mixed. To simplify the process, use a blender.
4. Divide the mixture into 8 servings.
5. Refrigerate for at least 4 hours or better at night.
6. Before serving, add whipped cream on top and sprinkle with grated chocolate without sugar.

- Chocolate Cake Espresso

Recipe

- 1 cup shredded dark chocolate (minimum 80% cocoa)
- 1 1/2 tsp vanilla extract
- 1/4 tsp salt

- 1/2 cup erythritol, powdered stevia, or another keto sweetener
- 1/2 cup unsweetened cocoa powder
- 1 tbsp freshly brewed and chilled espresso
- 3 large eggs

Cooking

1. Preheat the oven to 190 degrees and grease a round baking dish with unsalted butter. Put parchment on top and sprinkle it with a non-stick spray.
2. Put the pieces of dark chocolate in the microwave and heat for 1 minute. Stir and microwave again until the chocolate melts and becomes homogeneous.
3. Add eggs and sweetener to a large bowl. Beat with a blender or mixer at high speed for 1-2 minutes until light and foamy. Add cocoa powder and espresso, and beat until smooth.
4. Pour the batter into the pan. Smooth the top with a spatula. Bake for 18-20 minutes. Remove the cake from the oven and let it cool for 10 minutes.
5. Drag the knife along the edges of the cake to separate it from the mold. Put a large plate on the form upside down and quickly turn the cake on a plate. Remove and discard parchment paper.
6. Let the cake cool completely and refrigerate overnight. Garnish with berries if desired.

- Chocolate Orange Cupcake

Recipe

- 1 chopped orange
- 4 eggs, protein separated from yolks
- 1/2 cup low-carb sweetener
- 192 g almond flour
- 43 g unsweetened cocoa powder
- 1 tsp baking powder
- 1/2 tsp salt

Cooking

1. Put slices of orange in a pan and fill with water. Bring to a boil and cook for 1 hour. The orange should be soft enough to be pierced with a fork.
2. Pull out the orange and cool slightly.
3. Preheat the oven to 170 degrees.
4. Put slices of orange in a food processor and beat in mashed potatoes without lumps.
5. Add almond flour, cocoa powder, a low-carb sweetener, salt, baking powder, and egg yolks. Mix well.
6. Beat the egg whites until foam and carefully pour into the orange dough.
7. Place the dough in a greased cake pan.
8. Bake for 1 hour until cooked.

- Coconut Ice Cream with Berries

Recipe

- 476 g butter whipped cream
- 226 g coconut milk
- 100 g of erythritol
- 3 egg yolks
- 4.93 g vanilla extract
- 155 g berries
- 40 g sugar-free coconut flakes
- 29.57 g of vodka (optional)

Cooking

1. Heat cream and coconut milk in a saucepan over medium heat for about 3-5 minutes. Do not let the mixture boil!
2. While the cream is warming, beat the eggs, vanilla, and erythritol together.
3. Remove the cream from the heat and carefully pour it into the egg mixture. Beat until smooth.
4. Pour this mixture back into the pan over medium heat and beat for 5-10 minutes until the mixture begins to thicken slightly.
5. Remove from heat, add vodka and mix (if desired). Allow cooling.

6   Add the berries and coconut, then put the ice cream in an airtight container and place in the freezer. Take out the container every 30 minutes and mix the ice cream thoroughly. This may take about 4-5 hours.

- **Cranberry Low Carb Cookies**

Recipe

- 56 g coconut flour
- 60 g soft cream cheese
- 1 egg
- 113 g unsalted butter (soft)
- 113 g low carbohydrate erythritol
- 1 tsp vanilla extract
- 2 tsp cinnamon
- 1/2 tsp baking powder
- 1/2 tsp salt
- 110 g cranberries
- 43 g low sugar chocolate chips

Cooking

1   Preheat the oven to 180 degrees.
2   Combine butter, cream cheese, and erythritol.
3   Add vanilla extract and egg. Beat until smooth.
4   Add coconut flour, baking powder, cinnamon, and salt, and beat until smooth.
5   Add cranberries and chocolate chips.

6. With wet hands, grab a large ball the size of a walnut and place on a baking sheet with parchment paper.
7. Press the top of the ball with your hand or the back of the spoon to shape the cookies. Repeat the process (you should get about 15 pcs.).
8. Bake for 20 minutes until solid and golden.

- Cherry and poppy seed muffins

Ingredient

DRY

- 1 cup (120 g) raw buckwheat flour
- 1 ¼ cup oatmeal (155 g) oatmeal
- 2 tablespoons poppy seeds
- 2 teaspoons cinnamon
- ½ teaspoon cardamom
- 2 teaspoons baking powder

Wet

- 10 chopped figs

- A little more than 1 cup (260 ml) of vegetable milk, without sugar
- 2 ripe bananas
- 2 heaped tablespoons unsweetened applesauce
- 2 tablespoons peanut butter
- 1 pinch of sea salt (optional)
- ½ cup (50 g) dark chocolate (at least 70% cocoa), chopped
- 24 fresh or frozen cherries

Preparation

1. Preheat the oven to 355 ° F (180 ° C).
2. Cut the figs and soak them in the vegetable milk for at least half an hour. If you soak them more, place them in the fridge.
3. While the figs are soaking, finely chop the chocolate and set aside. Combine all other dry ingredients in a bowl. Place the figs and milk in the blender. Add all remaining wet ingredients and mix until smooth.
4. Pour the wet mixture over the dry ingredients and mix well. Make sure there are no lumps. Now add the chopped chocolate.
5. Fill molds 12 muffins (I molds using silicone) with the mass and finally hits two cherries on each muffin.
6. Bake for 25 to 30 minutes. Let them cool a little before trying to remove them from the molds.

- Homemade granola

Ingredient

- 3 cups flaked oatmeal
- ¼ cup chopped raw nuts
- ¼ cup raw pecans, chopped
- ¼ cup raw almonds, chopped
- ½ cup pure maple syrup
- 2 teaspoons vanilla
- 2 teaspoons cinnamon
- 1 pinch of salt (optional)

Process

1. Preheat the oven to 250-300 ° F (149 ° C).
2. Put all ingredients in a bowl, mix well, and cover everything with maple syrup. Spread the mixture on a baking sheet or broiler pan.
3. Bake for 30-40 minutes with occasional stirring until the mixture turns brown. Move the top plate to the wire rack and let it cool completely. Refrigerate the granola in a sealed jar.

- Tofu cashew cheesecake dessert

Ingredient

For The Mass

- 1 cup soaked cashews
- 6 ounces (175 g) of soft tofu
- 1 tablespoon peanut butter
- 1 small banana
- A handful of grated coconut
- 1 pinch of sea salt
- 1 ounce (30 ml) of water
- 2 tablespoons raw cocoa powder (mix it in half the dough)

The Swirl

- 1 tablespoon peanut butter
- 1 teaspoon agave syrup

End Mix

- 3 tablespoons of raisins, dipped in rum
- 4 chopped figs

Preparation

1. Soak the raisins in rum (not mandatory). (Of course, discard rum from children's containers). Soak the cashews in water for 2 to 2.5 hours. Rinse and drain.
2. Enter the dough ingredients (except cocoa powder) in the blender. Mix them until a uniform dough forms.
3. Now, put half of the mixture in a bowl and add the cocoa powder to the remaining half in the blender.

4 Mix half of the raisins and chopped figs in the brown dough and the other half in the white dough.
5 Prepare the swirl by mixing peanut butter (at room temperature) and agave syrup.
6 Now, start compiling the containers. Put the brown and white dough in the bowls in turns. Add small balls of butter mixture everywhere.
7 When you reach the last layer, add about 5 peanut butter balls on top. Now, it's all about your creativity and artistic skills. Take a sushi stick and make some cute swirls on top of the dessert.
8 Place the desserts in the fridge for a few hours. Cover the containers with foil if you need to keep them longer.

- Christmas nut cake with ginger

Ingredient

MASS MIX

- ½ cup unroasted buckwheat
- ½ cup of millet
- ⅓ cup (80 ml) unsweetened oat milk
- 1 ripe banana
- 1 tablespoon peanut butter
- 1 pinch of sea salt

- ½ teaspoon of turmeric
- ½ to 1 teaspoon of gingerbread spices
- 2 tablespoons baking powder (add them at the end)

TO COMBINE WITH MIXED MASS

- ¼ cup chopped hazelnuts
- ¼ cup chopped almonds
- ¼ cup chopped walnuts
- ¼ cup dried apricots, chopped
- ¼ cup raisins dipped in rum
- 5 chopped figs
- ⅛ cup goji berries
- 2 tablespoons grated orange peel or sugary orange peel (use organic)
- ¼ cup 50g (1.8oz) dark chocolate, chopped

Process

- Soak millet and buckwheat overnight (or throughout the day) in water in separate containers. Clean and drain them (you can use a strainer).
- Soak the raisins in a mixture of rum and hot water (half and a half) overnight. You can discard the soaking liquid later, or you can replace it with some of the oat milk in the recipe.
- Chop everything that needs to be cut from the second table.

- Heat the oven to 350 ° F (177 ° C) and line a bread pan with baking paper.
- Place the ingredients in the mixed dough, except for the baking powder, in a blender, and mix them until a uniform dough forms. Do not worry; It is supposed to be quite liquid since millet inflates considerably.
- Now, add the baking powder.
- Finally, combine (DO NOT LIQUUS) chopped nuts, dried fruits, and chocolate.
- Pour the dough into a bread pan and bake for 40 to 45 minutes until your Christmas cake is golden brown.
- Let cool before cutting and serving. If you leave the mold on the counter, cover it with a clean dishcloth or foil (loosely) to keep the cake moist.

CHAPTER ELEVEN

Mediterranean snacks recipes

- Grilled scallop top in cherry salmorejo

Ingredients

- 12 scallops
- 650 gr mature tomatoes
- 350 gr Cherries (I had frozen)
- 200 g milled bread from the day before
- 150 ml extra virgin olive oil Salt to taste
- 1/2 tooth Garlic

Preparations

1. We are going to make this cherry salmorejo, replacing part of the tomatoes of the classic salmorejo recipe with cherries. It is preferable that you use dark, very ripe cherries that bring a lot of flavors and enough color to the salmorejo, so that the change is noticed (I had a few frozen and boneless)
2. The first thing to do is chop the tomatoes and crush them. If we want to include cucumber in the recipe, we also add it by putting it in the blender glass. Then we will pass the result through a fine strainer, leaving it in a bowl, so it will not be necessary to remove the seeds or peel the tomatoes.
3. As for the cherries, we remove the peduncle and remove the seed with a sharp knife or with a boner. Once we have the pulp of cherries, we crush it and add it to the bowl. Add the sliced bread and let it moisten and soften.
4. Finally, we add the olive oil and optionally half a clove of garlic. Crush the whole and rectify salt.

Coconut snacks

Ingredient

- 1 cup pineapple juice
- 2 cups diced mango
- 2 ripe bananas, diced
- ½ vanilla branch
- 4 cups shredded coconut
- ¾ cup roasted grated coconut

Preparation

1. In a small pot, cook pineapple juice, mango, bananas, and vanilla over medium-low heat for 5 minutes.
2. Scrape the seeds of the vanilla branch in the pot and discard the branch; then cook them for two more minutes.
3. Put the ingredients that are in the pot and the 4 cups of grated coconut inside a food processor with an "S" shaped leaf and process them until you get a mixture without lumps, but firm.
4. Let the mixture cool for about 1 to 2 hours, then, using a small scoop for ice cream or a spoon, place a small amount in your hands and make a ball before rolling it over the toasted coconut.
5. Repeat the process until all your coconut snacks are rolled, I bet you can't eat just one!

Cucumber and kale open sandwich

Ingredient

- 2 slices of whole-grain bread, toasted
- 2 to 3 tablespoons of hummus prepared without tahini or oil
- 1 chopped green onion
- ¼ cup chopped fresh cilantro
- 2 medium kale leaves, chopped into small bite-sized pieces (about the size of coriander leaves)
- ½ small cucumber
- Mustard of your choice
- Lemon pepper (Mrs. Dash and Frontier brands have no salt)

Preparation

1. Spread hummus generously on toasted bread. Sprinkle the green onion, cilantro, and kale evenly over the hummus.
2. Slice the cucumber in 8 circles and spread each with a thin layer of mustard.
3. Place the cucumber slices, with the mustard down, on top of the coriander and kale layer and press down, if necessary, so that they remain in place.
4. Sprinkle the open sandwich generously with lemon pepper, cut it in half or quarters, if desired, and serve.

- Baked zucchini in cheese breading with aioli sauce

Recipe

Zucchini:

- 2 medium zucchini
- 2 eggs
- ⅓ cup grated parmesan
- 1 tbsp almond flour
- 1/4 tsp garlic powder
- 1 tsp dry parsley
- ½ tsp sea salt
- 1/4 tsp black pepper

Aioli sauce:

- 1/4 cup low-carb mayonnaise
- 1 clove of garlic
- 1 tsp fresh lemon juice
- 1/4 tsp black pepper
- A pinch of sea salt

Cooking

1. Preheat the oven to 204 degrees.
2. Cut the zucchini into strips.
3. Beat the eggs in a medium bowl.

4. In a separate bowl, mix grated parmesan, almond flour, garlic powder, dried parsley, sea salt, and black pepper.
5. Dip slices of zucchini in beaten eggs, and then in the cheese-almond mixture.
6. Place the coated slices on a wire rack placed on a baking sheet. Leave in the preheated oven for 20-25 minutes until they turn golden.
7. In a small bowl, mix all the ingredients for aioli.
8. Remove the zucchini from the oven and serve immediately.

- Stuffed Eggs with Cheese and Olives

Recipe

- 4 eggs
- 3 tbsp sour cream
- 1 tsp mustard
- 33.75 g black olives (finely chopped)
- 33.75 g blue cheese (crumbled)
- 1/4 tsp sea salt
- 1/8 tsp black pepper
- 1 tsp finely chopped dill, for garnish

Cooking

1. Put the eggs in a pot of cold water and bring to a boil. Cook for 10-12 minutes, and then clean them.
2. Hard-boiled eggs, cut in half lengthwise, remove the yolks in a bowl and soften them with a fork.
3. In the same bowl, add sour cream, mustard, sea salt and black pepper, and mix well until a creamy condition is obtained.
4. Add finely chopped olives and crumbled blue cheese.
5. Fill the egg whites with the prepared mixture using a pastry bag or bag / rolled parchment with a hole.
6. Arrange the boiled eggs on a plate, garnish with chopped dill and serve.

Apple "Halloween" lamps

What you will need

- 6 red apples
- 1 cup peanut butter
- 1 tablespoon date paste
- ½ teaspoon of pumpkin pie spice
- 1 cup of oil-free granola

Process

1. Preheat the oven to 300-350 ° F (177 ° C).
2. Cut the top of each apple.

3. Take out the inside with a spoon or a melon. Make sure the walls are thick.
4. Carefully carve the face of the flashlight to make eyes and mouth.
5. Melt peanut butter in a saucepan until smooth and smooth.
6. In a bowl, combine melted peanut butter with date paste and pumpkin spices.
7. Fill the apples with the peanut butter mixture and replace the apple tops.
8. Bake the apples on a baking sheet for 10 minutes.
9. Place the granola in the apples and bake for another 10 minutes.
10. Serve immediately.

- Mediterranean recipe of toasted chickpeas

Ingredients

- 15-ounce cans of chickpeas
- tablespoons of extra virgin olive oil
- teaspoons of red wine vinegar
- 2 teaspoons of fresh lemon juice
- 1 teaspoon kosher salt

- 1 teaspoon dried oregano
- 1/2 teaspoon garlic powder
- 1/2 teaspoon broken black pepper

Manual

1. Preheat the oven to 425 degrees and line a parchment paper baking sheet. Drain the chickpeas, rinse and dry thoroughly, then lay them in a layer on the baking sheet.
2. Roast for 10 minutes, then take out of the oven, turn the chickpeas with a spatula so that they bake evenly, and then roast for another 10 minutes.
3. Place the remaining ingredients in a large mixing bowl and whisk. Stir in the hot chickpeas and shake gently back and forth until completely covered.
4. Put the coated chickpeas back on the baking sheet and roast for another 10 minutes. Occasionally make sure that they do not overcook and burn. Let yourself cool down and enjoy it!

- Bean salad

Ingredients

- 1 pound 15 bean soup mix, dry bean mix
- 1 liter of grapes or cherry tomatoes, halved
- 1 cup of fresh or frozen corn

- 3/4 cup diced red pepper
- 1/2 cup diced red onion
- 1/2 cup chopped shallots
- 1/4 cup chopped parsley or cilantro
- 1/4 cup of olive oil
- spoons of balsamic vinegar
- tablespoons of rice vinegar
- 1 tbsp honey
- 1 tablespoon of Dijon mustard
- 1/2 teaspoon ground cumin
- salt and pepper

Instructions

1. The bean mix bag is opened and the seasoning pack discarded, if included. Soak and cook the beans as indicated on the box. Drain into a large bowl and put it in it.
2. While the beans cool, whisk the olive oil together in a small bowl, all tablespoons of vinegar, honey, mustard, cumin, 1 teaspoon salt and 1/2 teaspoon ground black pepper. Deposit aside.
3. Pour over the beans, all the chopped vegetables and herbs. Drizzle with the vinaigrette, then toss to cover well. Good taste, then salt and pepper if necessary. Cover and refrigerate until ready for serving.

- Spicy red lentil dip.

Ingredients

- 1 cup of collected and rinsed red lentils
- teaspoons of curry powder
- 1 teaspoon onion powder
- 1 teaspoon of sea salt
- 1/4 teaspoon black pepper
- 1/4 teaspoon turmeric
- 1/2 teaspoon of Garam Masala
- 1/2 teaspoon cumin
- Crackers to serve

Preparations

1. Put the red lentils and enough water in a saucepan to cover them 1 inch.
2. Bring to boil, then heat down to medium heat.
3. Let cook until soft, for 15-20 minutes.
4. If you still have water left, drain it.
5. Crush the lentils with a fork (they should be quite soft already).
6. Pour in the spices and whisk.
7. Warmly serve with crackers.

- Coconut Bars with Nuts

Recipe

- 60 g macadamia nuts
- 125 g almond oil
- 54.5 g coconut oil
- 6 tbsp unsweetened grated coconut
- 20 drops of stevia

Cooking

1. Grind macadamia nuts using a food processor or manually
2. Combine almond oil, coconut oil and grated coconut. Add macadamia nuts and stevia drops.
3. Thoroughly mix and pour the dough into a baking dish lined with parchment paper.
4. Refrigerate overnight, and then cut into pieces.

- Spinach Cheese Bread

Ingredients

- 225 g almond flour
- 2 tsp baking powder
- ½ tsp salt
- 100 g soft butter

- 85 g fresh spinach, chopped
- 1 clove garlic, finely chopped
- 1 tbsp chopped rosemary
- 2 large eggs
- 140 g grated cheddar cheese

Cooking

1. Preheat the oven to 200 degrees.
2. Put the almond flour, baking powder and salt in a large bowl. Mix well, then add oil and mix again.
3. Add the remaining ingredients (if you wish, you can leave a little cheddar for the top of the bread). Mix well.
4. Put the dough in a cast-iron skillet, greased with oil, and form a pancake with a thickness of about 3.5-4 cm.
5. Bake for 25-30 minutes; then leave the bread in the pan for 15 minutes to cool.

- Roasted Chickpeas

Ingredient

- 2 cans of 15 ounces (425 g) of chickpeas, rinsed and drained
- 1 teaspoon garlic powder
- 2 teaspoons chili powder

- ½ teaspoon of sea salt
- 2 tablespoons lemon juice

Process

1. Preheat the oven to 400 ° F (200 ° C). Line a baking sheet with parchment paper and set it aside.
2. Place the chickpeas in a one-gallon (liter) sealed plastic bag and add seasonings. Shake well until completely covered.
3. Spread spicy chickpeas evenly over the prepared baking sheet.
4. Bake for 45 to 55 minutes, stirring every 15 to 20 minutes so that the chickpeas cook evenly, until golden brown.
5. Serve hot or cold for a snack at any time.

- Almond butter toast with sweet potatoes and blueberries

Ingredient

- 1 sweet potato, sliced half a centimeter thick
- ¼ cup almond butter
- ½ cup blueberries

Preparation

1. Preheat the oven to 350-360 ° F (177 ° C).

2. Place the sweet potato slices on baking paper. Bake until soft, approximately 20 minutes. (You can also cook them in a toaster, but you would need to activate it at high temperature for three or four cycles).
3. Serve hot, coat with peanut butter and cranberries. Store any leftover sweet potato slices, without dressings, in an airtight container inside the refrigerator for a week. Reheat them in a toaster or in a toaster oven and cover them as instructed.

CONCLUSION

The Mediterranean diet is not exactly a diet, but a diet. In the Mediterranean diet there is no calorie count, no fasting and no elimination of whole food groups. The main idea is good balance and moderation. Balance your food intake well and emphasize those that can be consumed in abundance. Don't overdo it - prepare small portions and consume in moderation.

Everyone should think about how the Mediterranean diet can best be tailored to their lifestyle and personal taste. Focus your menu on the foods this diet contains and focus on the foods you like the most. Sweet treats are not excluded, but it is desirable that they are consumed less frequently and in smaller quantities.

Be physically active by aiming for at least 30 minutes a day or 150 minutes a week. Maintain a healthy weight. Drink alcohol in moderation and give up cigarettes.